The Art
of
Effective
Fracture
Fixation
with
Rush Pins

The Art
of
Effective
Fracture
Fixation
with
Rush Pins

F. Robert Brueckmann, M.D., F.A.C.S.
Orthopaedics-Indianapolis, Inc.
Methodist Hospital
Clinical Professor Orthopaedic Surgery
Indiana University
Indianapolis, Indiana

1990
Thieme Medical Publishers, Inc., NEW YORK
Georg Thieme Verlag, STUTTGART • NEW YORK

Thieme Medical Publishers, Inc.
381 Park Avenue South
New York, New York 10016

THE ART OF EFFECTIVE FRACTURE FIXATION WITH RUSH PINS
F. Robert Brueckmann

Library of Congress Cataloging-in-Publication Data

Brueckmann, F. Robert.
The art of effective fracture fixation with Rush pins.
1. Intramedullary fracture fixation.   I. Title.
[DNLM: 1. Bone Nails.   2. Fracture fixation, Intra-
medullary—methods. WE 185 B889a]
RD103.I53B78   1989   617.1'5   89-20461
ISBN 0-86577-323-8 (Thieme Medical Publishers)

Important note: Medicine is an ever-changing science. Research and clinical experience are continually broadening our knowledge, in particular our knowledge of proper treatment and drug therapy. Insofar as this book mentions any dosage or applications, readers may rest assured that the authors, editors, and publishers have made every effort to ensure that such references are strictly in accordance with the state of knowledge at the time of production of the book. Nevertheless, every user is requested to carefully examine the manufacturers' leaflets accompanying each drug to check on his own responsibility whether the dosage schedules recommended therein or the contraindications stated by the manufacturers differ from the statements made in the present book. Such examination is particularly important with drugs that are either rarely used or have been newly released on the market.

Some of the product names, patents, and registered designs referred to in this book are in fact registered trademarks or proprietary names even though specific reference to this fact is not always made in the text. Therefore, the appearance of a name without designation as proprietary is not to be construed as a representation by the publisher that it is in the public domain.

Printed in the United States of America.

5 4 3 2

TMP ISBN 0-86577-323-8
GTV ISBN 3-13-741501-2

To my parents, friends, colleagues and teachers who encouraged my efforts. Most of all to my wife, Betty Lee, who has enriched my life.

Contents

Preface

I first became interested in the use of pin fixation in 1961, after reading Dr. Rush's *Atlas of Rush Pin Technics.* At that time, most femoral shaft fractures were treated in traction, intra-articular fractures were treated in casts, and metal was never used in compound wounds. Intramedullary fixation was in its infancy. Available in the late 1960s, the portable image intensifier made closed and semi-open pinnings easy, especially with a pin that could be twisted to reduce the fracture from a distance.

Because of the many problems associated with fracture healing and infection, the period of screw fixation to treat shaft fractures quickly passed. Reamed intramedullary fixation became a more acceptable method to use with femoral shaft fractures, but was limited because of the anatomic limitations of isthmic fractures. Fortunately, the development and effective use of Rush pin fixation techniques occurred at this time.

The results of Rush pin procedures are equal to or better than the current reamed procedures. The basic principles of static or dynamic fixation techniques easily can be used in all long bone fractures. New instruments and implants do not need to be available for new fracture situations. Rush pins provide a simple and efficient method of fracture treatment. This text has been written and organized to aid the practicing orthopaedic surgeon in pin fixation.

F. Robert Brueckmann, M.D.

Acknowledgments

I greatly appreciate the efforts of the many contributors who assisted in the development of this book. I would specifically like to thank the following individuals and groups of people.

Clyde B. Kernek, M.D., for his clear description of bone healing with intramedullary fixation. Dr. Kernek's interest in basic bone healing, as well as his active clinical teaching responsibilities within the Indiana University Orthopaedic Program, have been stimulating to me.

Brenda Q. Kester, medical illustrator, from the Medical Media Production Department at Methodist Hospital of Indiana, Inc. She always handled the revisions with a friendly smile, and her multiple illustrations were done with the highest quality of workmanship.

Stephen J. Jay, M.D., and the division of Academic Affairs at Methodist Hospital of Indiana, Inc. Their support and encouragement are greatly appreciated.

The Berivon Comany, for their permission for unrestricted use of materials from *Atlas of Rush Pin Technics*, for their production of fracture table modifications, and for the use of instruments and implants for teaching purposes.

Finally, I thank Thieme Medical Publishers, Inc., for the diligence accorded to this book regarding its contents, editing, and printing.

CHAPTER 1

History

1907—Lambotte:
  Intramedullary Tacks
1937—Rush:
  Round Intramedullary Pin
1940—Küntscher:
  V-shaped Intramedullary Nail
1947—Hanson-Street:
  Diamond-shaped Nail
1949—Rush:
  Round Resilient Intramedullary Pin
1950—Küntscher:
  Cloverleaf Intramedullary Nail
1951—Lottes:
  Precurved Triangular Tibial Nail
1968—Schneider:
  X-shaped Intramedullary Nail

Albin Lambotte of Belgium was undoubtedly the father of modern osteosynthesis, for in 1907, he pinned the clavicle with a thin metal device, used intramedullary tacks, and later wrote a book on the surgical treatment of fractures in 1913. Hey Groves, in 1918, in a report on war injuries, demonstrated three cases of fractures of the femur treated with a perforated steel tube, a cross-shaped steel rod, and a solid, round steel rod used for intramedullary fixation. In 1937, Leslie V. Rush, Sr., and H. L. Rush reported a case of intramedullary fixation for a Monteggia fracture.[1]

In 1940, Gerhard Küntscher of Berlin reported on a V-shaped intramedullary nail used to treat fractures of the femoral shaft. In 1950 he redesigned a cloverleaf-shaped nail, and in 1952 introduced medullary reaming. By 1947, Dana Street and Harvey Hanson of the Campbell Clinic reported on a new diamond-shaped nail for intramedullary fixation of the femur. By 1949, Leslie V. Rush, Sr., and H. L. Rush reported on the evolution of medullary fixation by a longitudinal pin and a "medullary pin for spring-type fixation as applied to the femur."[2]

The discovery by W. C. Roentgen in 1895 of special rays that would penetrate the body and leave a shadow on a photographic plate made the diagnosis and the treatment of fractures more exact. With the development of image intensification x rays, intramedullary fixation became a practical method for surgeons in the care of fractures. The portable intraoperative image intensifier that has retention devices to hold the images, without continued radiation to the patient or the surgeon, is standard now. Others, including W. Schneider in 1968, J. O. Lottes in 1951, and L. Bohler and J. Bohler in 1949, reported the use of medullary fixation devices but were without the benefits of image intensification. Since image intensification has been possible, S. T. Hansen and A. Winquist and M. W. Chapman have been advocates of closed intramedullary nailing of the fractured femur.

In the early 1960s, Donald S. Blackwell and I visited Leslie V. Rush (Fig. 1—1) in Meridian, Mississippi, and were impressed with the rapidity of healing of femoral fractures treated in this manner. The majority of the cases and the experience presented here are the result of treating patients in Indianapolis at the Methodist Hospital of Indiana, Inc., and at the Marion County General Hospital (now Wishard Hospital), both active parts of the Indiana University School of Medicine Orthopedic Training Program. Cases presented in the study on femoral shaft fractures are from physicians who trained in the Indiana University program, the Methodist Hospital, and others, all of whom I consider my good friends.

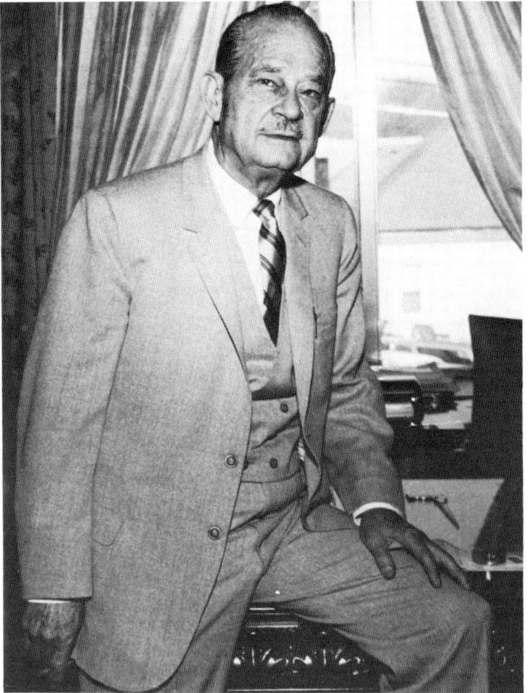

Figure 1—1.   Leslie V. Rush, Sr., M.D., born February 16, 1905, in Meridian, Mississippi, and died February 8, 1987.

REFERENCES

1. Rush, L.D., Rush, H.L.: A reconstruction operation for a comminuted fracture of the upper third of the ulna. Am. J. Surg. 38:332–333, 1937.
2. Rush, L.V., Rush, H.L.:A medullary fracture pin for spring-type fixation: as applied to the femur. Mississippi Doctor Sept:119–126, 1949.

SUGGESTED READINGS

Chapman, M.W.: The use of immediate internal fixation in open fractures. Orthop. Clin. North Am. 11:579, 1980.

Hansen, S.T., Jr., Winquist, R.A.: Closed intramedullary nailing of femur. Clin. Orthop. 138:56–61, 1979.

Küntscher, G.: Die marknagelung von knockenbrucken. Arch. Klin. Chir. 200:443–455, 1940.

Rush, L.V.: Atlas of Rush Pin Technics. Meridian, Mississippi, The Berivon Company, 1955.

Street, D.M., Funk, K.: One hundred fractures of the femur treated by means of a diamond shaped medullary nail.: J. Bone Joint Surg. 33:649, 1951.

CHAPTER 2

Fracture Healing with Medullary Fixation

Clyde B. Kernek

THREE PHASES OF FRACTURE HEALING

Fracture healing has been divided into three phases. The first is the inflammatory phase, the second is the reparative phase, and the third is the remodeling phase.[1] The trauma that causes the fracture of bone also damages the circulation to the bone fragments at the fracture site, and necrosis of bone occurs.[2–4] Blood supply and osteogenic cells are basic to fracture healing; and both are damaged at the time of fracture. The degree of injury to bone and soft tissues depends on the amount of energy causing the fracture.

Inflammatory Phase

The inflammatory phase starts at the moment of fracture and includes soft-tissue injury to the periosteum and surrounding muscle, with injury to the circulation of these tissues as well as the bone. Hematoma forms at the fracture site, and osteocytes die at the ends of the bone fragments. There is vasodilatation in the fractured limb, and clinically this is observed as increased warmth, which extends into the reparative phase.

Reparative Phase

The reparative phase consists of organization of the fracture hematoma and the formation of the healing callus by the ingrowth of osteogenic cells and vascular supply. This callus is made up of fibrous, cartilaginous, and osseous tissues. The formation of external and internal callus increases the stability of the fracture fragments and eventually produces clinical union of the fracture. Brighton divided the reparative phase into the stage of soft callus and the stage of hard callus.[5]

Cells and blood supply are basic to fracture healing and the formation of callus. Injury to the osteogenic cell source and the blood supply can impair fracture healing. This injury includes not only the trauma causing the fracture, but also any subsequent injury from surgical management. Also, loss of bone can impair healing and may require bone grafting. Although adequate immobilization of the fractured bone is very important to healing, the formation of external callus is promoted by muscle activity, early weight-bearing, and a limited degree of motion.[6,7] Sarmiento and colleagues found that functional weight-bearing accelerates the rate of healing by allowing the callus to achieve mechanical adequacy for function faster than does non-weight-bearing.[8]

Remodeling Phase

The remodeling phase starts when the fracture has healed, as determined by clinical and radiographic evaluation.[5] In 1892, Wolff developed his law, which states that the skeletal system responds to the mechanical stress placed on it. The remodeling of the healed fracture follows Wolff's law. This phase continues on for years, based on radioisotope studies. Necrotic bone may be resorbed, become viable cancellous bone, or become viable cortical bone.[9]

The four biomechanical stages of fracture repair have been defined by White and associates.[10] Stage I (failure through the fracture site with a low level of stiffness) correlates with the reparative phase of fracture healing. Stage II (failure through the fracture site with a high level of stiffness), Stage III (failure partially through the fracture site and intact bone), and Stage IV (failure through intact bone) correlate with the progressive

increase in strength in the remodeling phase of fracture healing.

HEALING OF SHAFT FRACTURES

Shaft fractures treated by medullary fixation heal by the formation of external callus. This formation of external callus is affected by damage to the circulation of the cortical bone and soft tissues. Damage to circulation is caused by the injury trauma as well as any subsequent surgical trauma.[11] Insertion of a medullary device injures the medullary circulation initially. Circulation of diaphyseal bone is primarily centrifugal,[12] but there is evidence of dual circulation for cortical bone.[13–16] So periosteal circulation becomes very important with medullary fixation, and is not further damaged by closed medullary fixation. However, open medullary fixation by wide surgical exposure further damages periosteal circulation and causes more avascular cortex. The semi-open reduction described by Rush is a limited surgical exposure to minimize further surgical trauma and to preserve healing potential.[17] Medullary circulation does regenerate after medullary fixation, and with a loose-fitting pin the circulation regenerates rapidly to fill the areas not filled by the pin.[18,19]

Other factors affect the formation of external callus. The size of external callus is related to the amount of motion at the fracture site.[9] External callus forms more on the concave side of a fracture.[3] Muscle damage retards fracture healing.[20]

Radiographic patterns for the formation of external callus have been observed in closed fractures of the femoral shaft that were treated by closed and open medullary fixation with Rush pins.[21] The circulatory status at the fracture site may be a factor in these callus patterns. Closed pinning tends to form a more adequate lateral callus and to form smooth, dense callus (Fig. 2–1). Open

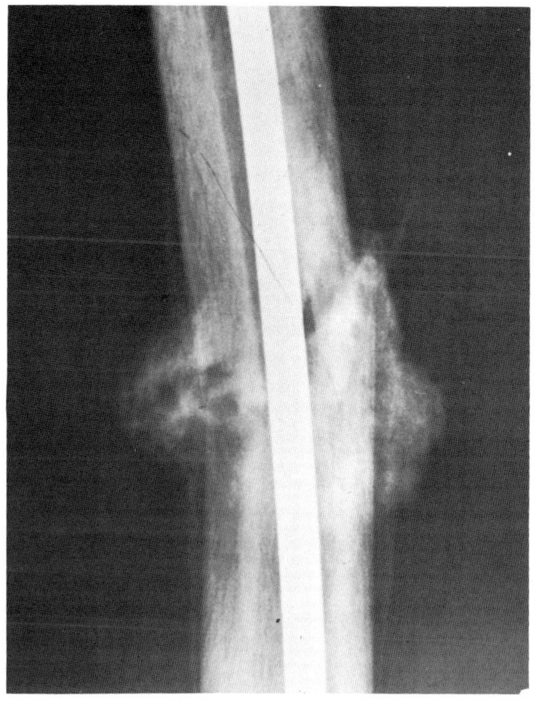

A

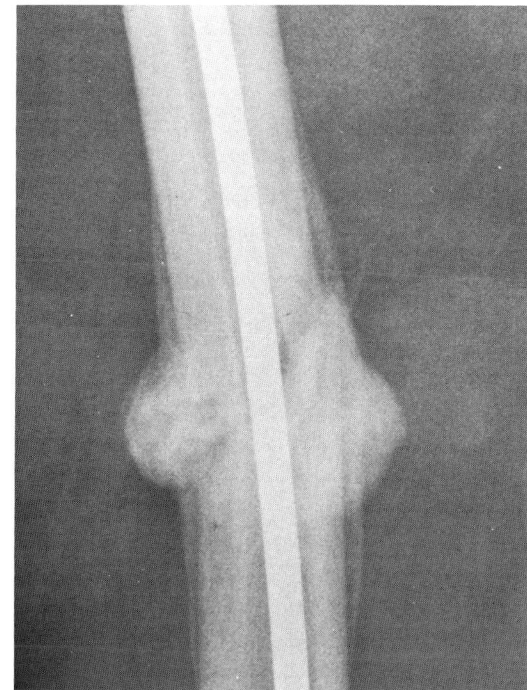

B

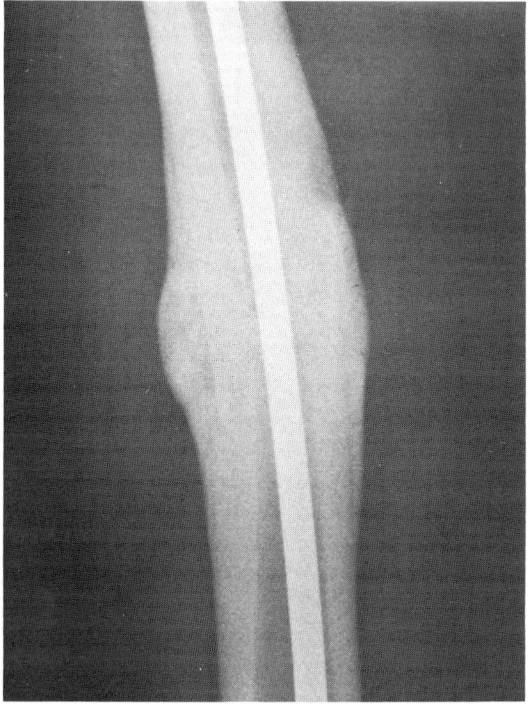

C

Figure 2–1. Closed fracture of right femur treated by closed Rush pin fixation. (**A**) Anteroposterior radiograph made at 2 months after pinning demonstrates early formation of callus in the lateral and medial parts. (**B**) Anteroposterior radiograph made at 3 months demonstrates smooth dense callus. (**C**) Anteroposterior radiograph made at 9 months demostrates remodeling of the femoral fracture.

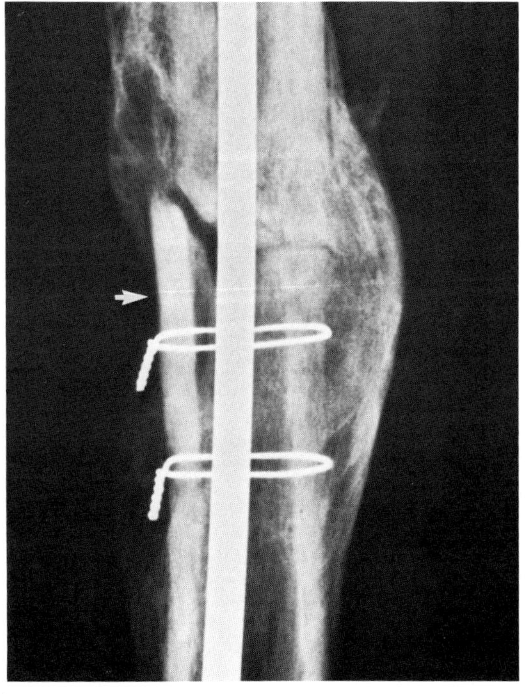

A

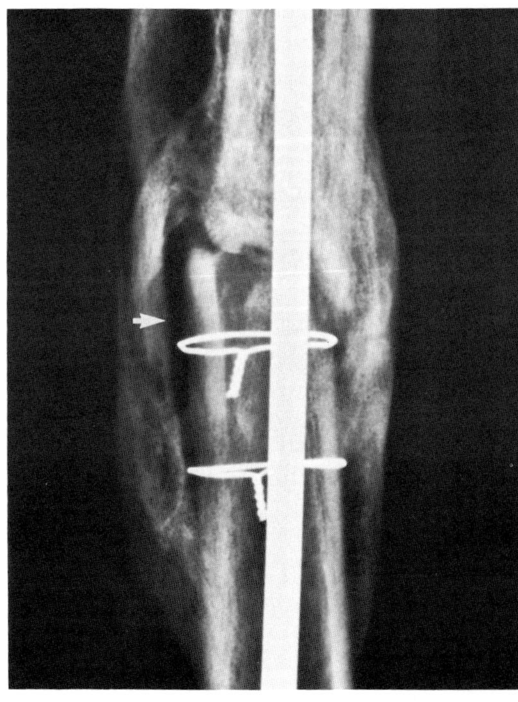

B

Figure 2–2.   Closed fracture of right femur treated by open reduction and internal fixation with a Rush pin and cerclage wire over a butterfly fragment. (**A**) The anteroposterior radiograph made at 5½ months after internal fixation demonstrates scant formation of callus over a segment of dense cortex (arrow), which represents avascular cortex, in the lateral part. (**B**) The lateral radiograph demonstrates callus in the posterior part with a radiolucent space (arrow) under the callus and over the wires and dense cortex.

less lateral callus, has more radiolucent space under the bridging callus over the cortex, and may cause exuberant callus with the appearance of myositis ossificans. The avascular cortex of shaft fractures (Fig. 2–2) may be identified by the radiographic findings of bridging callus with a radiolucent space under the callus, relative increased density of cortical bone, and resorption of cortical bone.

HEALING OF CANCELLOUS BONE

Metaphyseal and epiphyseal fractures generally involve cancellous bone, which has a good osteogenic cell source and blood supply. These fractures heal mainly by the formation of internal callus and heal more rapidly than shaft fractures. In addition to the internal callus of metaphyseal fractures, external callus may also be important in fractures, such as those in the supracondylar region of the femur. Shaft fractures involve cortical bone, which has a poorer cell source and blood supply than cancellous bone. Fractures of cancellous bone may occasionally be associated with interruptions of blood supply that would be expected to impair healing. Insertion of a medullary device would cause little additional injury to the circulation of metaphyseal and epiphyseal bone.

NONUNION

Unfortunately some fractures do not heal even with good management. Although the exact causes are not known, nonunion is associated with the following conditions.[1,22]

- Open fractures and loss of bone
- Comminuted fractures
- Segmental fractures
- Infection at the fracture site
- Pathologic fractures
- Fractures with poor blood supply
- Fractures with soft-tissue interposition
- Fractures held in distraction
- Inadequate immobilization
- Inadequate open reduction

When internal fixation is used to treat a fracture, the failure of union of the fracture may lead to ultimate failure of the implant.

REFERENCES

1. Cruess, R.L.: Healing of bone, tendon, and ligament, in Fractures in Adults, ed 2, edited by Rockwood, C.A., Jr., Green, D.P. Philadelphia, J. B. Lippincott, 1984, Vol 1, pp 147–159.
2. Ham, A.W., Cormack, D.H.: Histology, ed 8. Philadelphia, J. B. Lippincott, 1979, pp 450–451.
3. Sevitt, S.: Bone Repair and Fracture Healing in Man. Current Problems in Orthopaedics. New York, Churchill Livingstone, 1981. pp 66–67, 87.
4. McLean, F.C., Urist, M.R.: Bone: Fundamentals of the Physiology of Skeletal Tissue, ed 3. Chicago, University of Chicago Press, 1968, pp 222–223.
5. Brighton, C.T.: Principles of fracture healing. Part I, the biology of fracture repair, in American Academy of Orthopaedic Surgeons Instructional Course Lectures, edited by Murray, J.A. St. Louis, C. V. Mosby, 1984, vol 33, pp 61–62.
6. Dehne, E., Metz, C.W., Deffer, P.A., Hall, R.M.: Nonoperative treatment of the fractured tibia by immediate weight bearing. J. Trauma 1:514–535, 1961.
7. Sarmiento, A.: A functional below-the-knee cast for tibial fractures. J. Bone Joint Surg. 49A:855–875, 1967.
8. Sarmiento, A., Schaeffer, J.F., Beckerman, L., et al.: Fracture healing in rat femora as affected by functional weight-bearing. J. Bone Joint Surg. 59A:369–375, 1977.
9. McKibbin, B.: The biology of fracture healing in long bones. J. Bone Joint Surg. 60B:150–162, 1978.
10. White, A.A., III, Panjabi, M.M., Southwick, W.O.: The four biomechanical stages of fracture repair. J. Bone Joint Surg. 59A:188–192, 1977.
11. Küntscher, G.: The Callus-Problem, translated by Altner, P.C. St. Louis, Warren H. Green, 1974, p 44.
12. Brookes, M.: The Blood Supply of Bone. London, Butterworths, 1971, p 199.
13. Danckwardt-Lilliestrom, G.: Reaming of the medullary cavity and its effect on diaphyseal bone. Acta Orthop. Scand. 128 (suppl):135–143, 1969.
14. Trias, A., Fery, A.: Cortical circulation of long bones. J. Bone Joint Surg. 61A:1052–1059, 1979.
15. Weiland, A.J., Berggren, A., Jones, L.: The acute effects of blocking medullary blood supply on regional cortical blood flow in canine ribs as measured by the hydrogen washout technique. Clin. Orthop. 165:265–272, 1982.
16. Whiteside, L.A., Ogata, K., Lesker, P., et al.: The acute effects of periosteal stripping and medullary reaming on regional bone blood flow. Clin. Orthop. 131:266–272, 1978.
17. Rush, L.V.: Atlas of Rush Pin Technics, ed 2. Meridian, Mississippi, The Berivon Company, 1976, p 29.
18. Rhinelander, F.W.: Effects of medullary nailing on the normal blood supply of diaphyseal cortex, in American Academy of Orthopaedic Surgeons Instructional Course Lectures. St. Louis, C. V. Mosby, 1973, Vol 22, 161–187.
19. Rhinelander, F.W., Baragry, R.A.: Microangiography in bone healing. I. Undisplaced closed fractures. J. Bone Joint Surg. 44A:1273–1298, 1962.
20. Holden, C.E.A.: The role of blood supply to soft tissue in the healing of diaphyseal fractures. J. Bone Joint Surg. 54A:993–1000, 1972.
21. Kernek, C.B., Robb, J.A.: External callus formation of closed femoral shaft fractures treated by medullary fixation. Orthopedics 9:45–50, 1986.
22. Crenshaw, A.H.: Delayed union and nonunion of fractures, in Campbell's Operative Orthopaedics, ed 7, edited by Crenshaw, A.H. St. Louis, C. V. Mosby, 1987, vol 3, p 2053.

CHAPTER 3

Intramedullary Fixation

Universal Conditions for Fracture Fixation
Metal Properties of Resilient Pins
Causes for Nail or Pin Migration
Requirements of Intramedullary Fixation of Long Bones

According to Seligson, in his excellent text *Concepts in Intramedullary Nailing,* Küntscher listed four conditions for successful fracture fixations. He gave functional mobilization primary importance, saying, "First, fixation so that the fragments will not part;" second, "Healing of the incision as far away from the fracture as possible;" third, "favorable conditions for callus formation as in hip nailing;" fourth, "an overlooked requirement for simplicity and applicability to most common fractures."[1] His list differs from Danis' conditions, which included anatomic restoration.[2] Küntscher's doctrines have been popularized in part as the Association for the Study of the problems of internal fixation, (AO) principles.

Gerhard Küntscher purposely chose the word "nailing" for his method of fixation because of the similarity of pounding a nail into wood, which produces an expansion effect of elastic wood fibers. This gripping holds the nail in the wood. In the cloverleaf nail of Küntscher, the mechanism is in the reverse.

The development of the current Rush pin from intramedullary Steinmann pins and cerclage wires in 1937 has come with the development of metallurgical studies. Scientists of metallurgy developed various stainless steels, 316 and 316-L. Cast cobalt chrome alloys, wrought cobalt chrome alloys, and titanium and its alloys were also used in internal fixation devices. The mechanical properties of these metals are listed in Table 3-1.

With strain or work hardening there is an increase in hardness and strength caused by plastic deformation at temperatures lower than the recrystalization range of the metal. This produces a higher tensile strength, a greater yield strength, and a relatively low modulus of elasticity. It is the resiliency of the pin, the capacity of the 316L by virtue of high yield strength and low elastic modulus, to exhibit considerable elastic recovery on release of the load. The shape and the resiliency of the Rush pin, along with the insertion technique, produce the satisfactory end result in bone healing.

Fracture fixation by intramedullary techniques has a long list of potential complications from induced infection, nonunion of the fracture, and mechanical complications. The typical mechanical failures are migration, plastic bending, or fatigue fracture of the nail; delayed union

Table 3–1. Typical Mechanical Properties at Room Temperature

Type	Modulus of Elasticity (psi)	Yield Strength (psi)	Tensile Strength (psi)	% Elongation
316 LVM				
Annealed	28×10^6	75,000	30,000	40
Cold worked	28×10^6	100,000	125,000	12
Co-Cr-Mo	35×10^6	65,000	95,000	8
Cr-Cr-Ni-W	34×10^6	45,000	125,000	30
Ti	16×10^6	65,000	50,000	20
Ti-6Al-4V	16×10^6	115,000	125,000	10

LVM = type of stainless steel; Co = cobalt; Cr = chromium; Mo = molybdenum; Ni = nickel; W = tungsten; Ti = titanium; Al = aluminum; V = vanadium

Source: American Society of Testing Materials Designation F138-86, F75-87, F90-87, F67-88 F136-84.

or nonunion after intramedullary nailing may also be due to mechanical factors. Street and Funk,[3] in 1951, reported the end results of femoral nailing, with mechanical complications being bent nails (4.3%), broken nails (1.5%), and nonunion (4%). The rate of nail migration varies largely according to different authors. It appears that many of the broken and bent nails are related to failure of healing, and this corresponds with a similar rate of nonunion of the fracture. According to Marens, Frankel, and Burstein;[4] nail migration is caused by repeated angulation in the bending mode, and this was demonstrated in their experiments. Additional complications of intramedullary fixation are shortening, malrotation, and angulation of the bone and nerve palsy, due to either the position of the patient, traction devices, or direct injury.

For many years intramedullary fixation was delayed because of fear of fat embolism but Riska[5] and associates[4] and Winquist and Hansen[6] indicated that this is not the case and that early fixation is the treatment of choice. I have used this method of early fixation with gradually increasing frequency since the mid-1960s.

The basic requirements for intramedullary fixation of long-bone fractures are:

1. An available and patent medullary canal.
2. A reducible fracture so that the medullary canals can be continuous.
3. An intramedullary device that can be inserted and removed with proper instrumentation.

A patent medullary canal is usually seen in acute fractures but may be absent in:

1. Hypertrophic nonunions.
2. Intramedullary bone, that is or has been infected or diseased.
3. Iatrogenic defects caused by screws, prosthetic stems, or bone cement.
4. Childrens shaft bones protected by epiphyseal plates.

A reducible fracture, so that the medullary canals are continuous, may depend on:

1. Tubulation of comminuted fractures by wire cerclage.
2. Manipulation of displaced fracture ends that are held apart by shortening or by soft-tissue interposition.

Medullary filling nails, because of the varying diameters of the medullary canals, may need to have medullary canal reaming so that the nail can have as much purchase on both sides of the fracture to control rotation and provide stability. The requirements for intramedullary reaming are:

1. Access to the medullary canal in a relatively straight line.
2. A patent medullary canal.
3. Proper reaming instruments and insertion instruments.
4. Stabilization of segmental fractures prior to reaming if included in the fixation.

REFERENCES

1. Seligson, D. (ed.): Concepts in Intramedullary Nailing. Orlando, Florida, Grune and Stratton, 1985, p 14.
2. Danis, R.: Théorie et practique de l'osteosynthe. Paris: Masson & Cie. 1947.
3. Street, D.M., Funk, K.: One hundred fractures of the femur treated by means of a diamond shaped medullary nail. J. Bone Joint Surg. 33:649–669, 1951.
4. Martens, M., Frankel, V.H., Burstein, A.H.: Ultimate properties of intramedullary nails. Injury 4:18–24, 1972.
5. Riska, E.B., von Bonsdorff, H., Hakkinen, S. et al.: Prevention of fat embolism by early fixation of fractures in patients with multiple injuries. Injury 8:110–116, 1976.
6. Winquist, R.A., Hansen, S.T., Jr.: Closed intramedullary nailing of femoral shaft fractures. J. Bone Joint Surg. 66A:529–539, 1984.

Principles and Use of Basic Pin Techniques

Principles of effective fracture fixation with Rush pins are:

1. To protect the soft tissues surrounding the fracture to provide stability and preserve the blood supply.

2. To effectively immobilize the fracture by intramedullary fixation using three-point fixation, which only temporarily interferes with the intramedullary blood supply.

3. To promote the active use of the adjacent joints.

Muscle power is needed for effective immobilization at the fracture site. To rely on bone fixation alone is to consider only one part of the problem. Consider a television tower piercing the sky and visualize it as the bone of an extremity with its hollow core. The supporting guy wires attached at various heights provide its strength against the elements. Muscle and tendons are the equivalent of the guy wires and provide soft-tissue support for effective fracture fixation.

Radiographs of orthopaedic implants can be misleading since they always suggest static conditions. Orthopaedic surgeons constantly review radiographs of screws, plates, prostheses, and nails, assuming that they are static. Radiographs of Rush pins appear static but the pin function may be either static or dynamic. For example, radiographs of a supracondylar femoral fracture treated with Rush pins will show a gentle curve to the pins as they lie in the medullary canal. If the pins were static, they would have the same curve. Actually, when the pins are removed, they will be relatively straight, indicating the dynamic type of fixation present, due to the resiliency of the straight pin curving from the condyle into the distal end of the medullary canal.

Static type of fixation is present when precurved ¼-inch (6.35mm) pins are used. When removed, the pins are in the same curve; thus, the diameter of the pin, as well as the method of insertion, determine whether the action of the pin is dynamic or static. In all cases, the muscle pull across the fracture site induces a dynamic effect.

Long bones basically have a larger diameter at the articular ends and the narrowest diameter in the middle. The thinnest cortex is at the metaphyseal and epiphyseal ends and the thickest cortex is at the diaphysis. This situation is ideal

for pin insertion through a small incision; it leaves the soft tissues intact.

A curved pin in the same plane as a curved bone or a straight pin in a straight bone provides only static control and no rotational control, particularly if the pin is smaller in diameter than the medullary canal (Fig. 4–1). The muscle forces of the body provide a dynamic effect as they may create an angular force that must be resisted by the pin and the opposing muscle. The reduced fracture itself may provide stability, particularly when the enveloping muscles and soft tissues are present (Fig. 4–2). The interdigitating surfaces of a transverse fracture, when in compression from muscle spasm, are stable. The oblique and spiral fractures, when retubulated, become stable. The technique of passing the wire about the bone without stripping the periosteum is essential to prompt healing and stabilization.

The "vase of flowers" effect depicts the dynamic aspects of the resilient pin (Fig. 4–3). Flowers with flexed stems that are entered into a vase obliquely tend to upright themselves within the vase because of the resiliency of the stems which exert point pressure within the vase. A resilient rod introduced obliquely into the tubular cavity of a bone acts similarly. This principle has broad application and

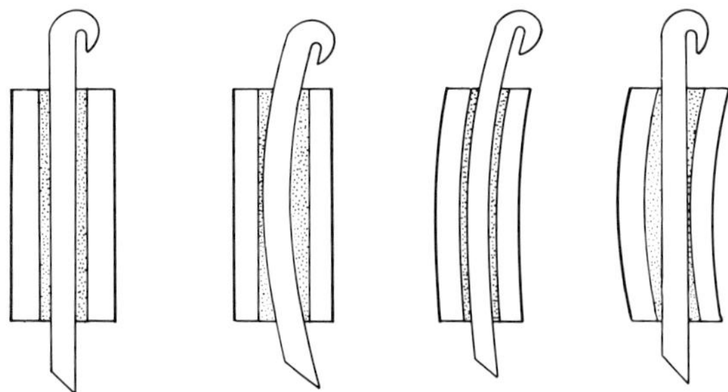

Figure 4–1. Influences of preshaping pin and bone contour. (**A**) A pin that is preshaped to the contour of the bone exerts no dynamic force. (**B**) A curved pin in a straight bone exerts pressure at three points. (**C**) A pin that is preshaped to the contour of the bone exerts no dynamic force. (**D**) A straight pin in a curved bone exerts pressure at three points.

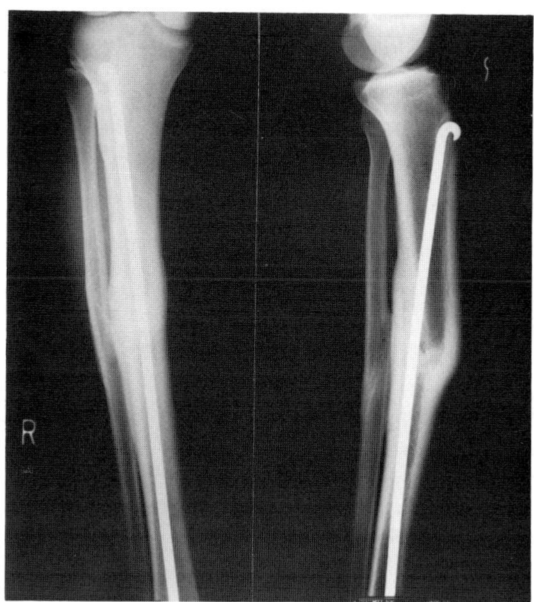

Figure 4–2. The tibia of a 20-year-old man, 1 year after fracture. A straight pin provides stability, but when it is inserted from the edge of a bone in a tibial shaft it tends to curve bone as seen here. A pre-shaped pin would prevent this, as well as control rotation.

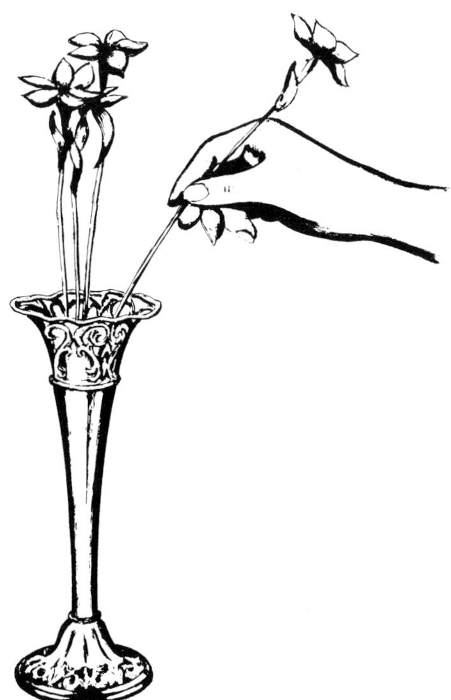

Figure 4–3. "Vase of flowers" effect depicts the dynamic aspects of the resilient pin.

is commonly used with supracondylar femoral fractures, condylar femoral fractures, Colles' fractures, and lateral malleolar fractures.

Fracture reduction is needed prior to fixation and is easiest when the fracture is fresh and there is adequate anesthesia. It is almost axiomatic that fractures that can be reduced can be pinned closed. Some fractures are so unstable that reduction is only possible with external force in addition to traction. From this comes the statement that the ability to temporarily reduce a fracture is tantamount to closed pinning.

Closed reduction of small bones is usually done by manual traction and large bones of the lower extremity, by traction, particularly with a fracture or extension table. The Rush fracture table developed by the Berivon Company works perfectly for fractures of the lower extremity. The foot plate can be sterilized but is seldom needed that way.

The next method of reduction is the semi-open technique (Fig. 4–4). This

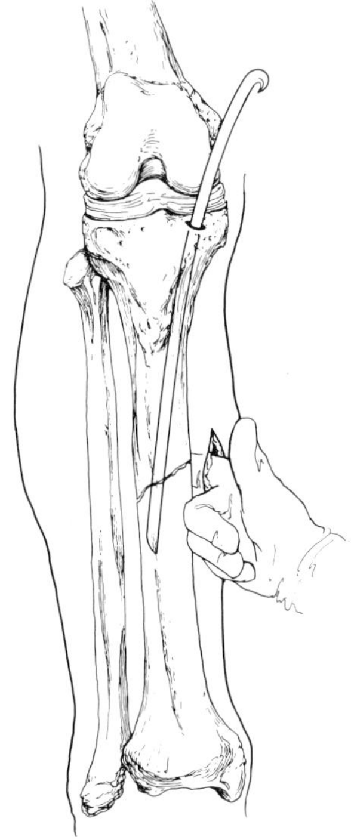

Figure 4–4. "Semi-open" technique.

method allows the surgeon to manipulate the bone with the fingers or instruments until the sled runner point of the pin can be placed across the fracture site. The fracture does not need to be visualized, stripped, or seen with anything other than the surgeon's finger.

Open reduction allows direct visualization of the fracture. This is usually done when bone grafting is needed or pathologic fractures require the use of polymethylmethacrylate cement. One must always preserve soft-tissue attachments by an appropriate surgical approach.

The sled runner point of the Rush pin can be used to manipulate the fracture with a closed or with the semi-open technique. The sled runner tip is manipulated by twisting the head of the pin. Prebending the pin in a gentle curve allows the radius of the point of the sled runner tip to be increased to the diameter of the bone at the fracture site. This greatly enhances the chance of a closed reduction of a fracture that could not be reduced completely by external manipulation (Figs. 4–5, 4–6).

To obtain the effect of the resiliency of the pin, it must be put into the bone at a proper angle so that the impaction of the pin in the bone bends the pin and allows the hooked end to cause a force to hold the fracture. To be effective, it obviously must oppose the muscular forces that cause deformity or the force of an opposite pin.

THE EXTENSION FRACTURE TABLE

The fracture table (Fig. 4–7) is used to put the affected limb in traction, usually without skeletal attachments, and in the supine position, to reduce fractures at the hip or of the femur, the supracondylar region of the femur, and the tibia, both the proximal part and the shaft, so that

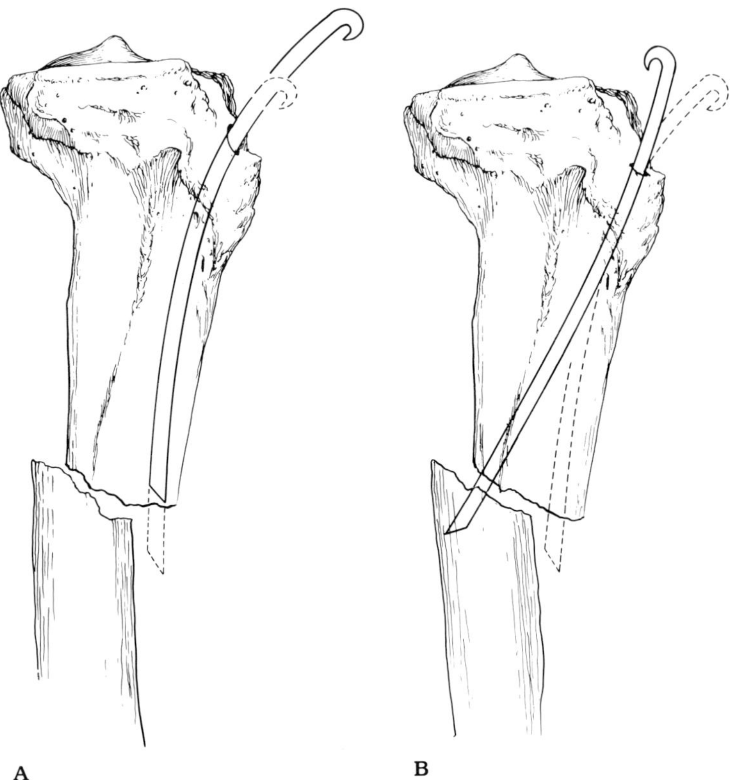

Figure 4–5. Reduction of fracture using a preshaped pin with sled runner tip. (A) Rotating a preshaped pin will allow passage of the pin into the distal fragment. (B) The pin is rotated back to the original insertion position and seated.

A   B

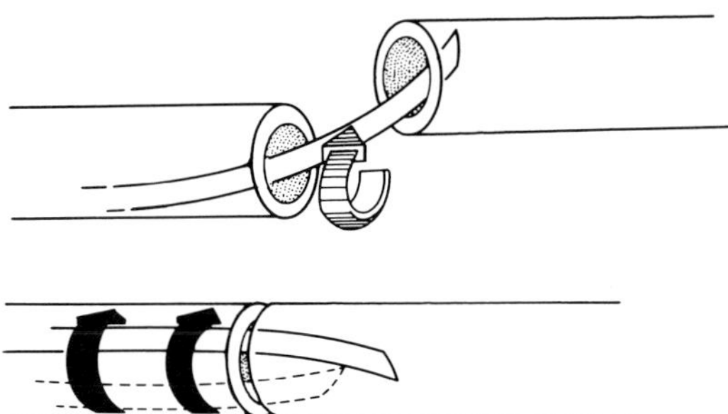

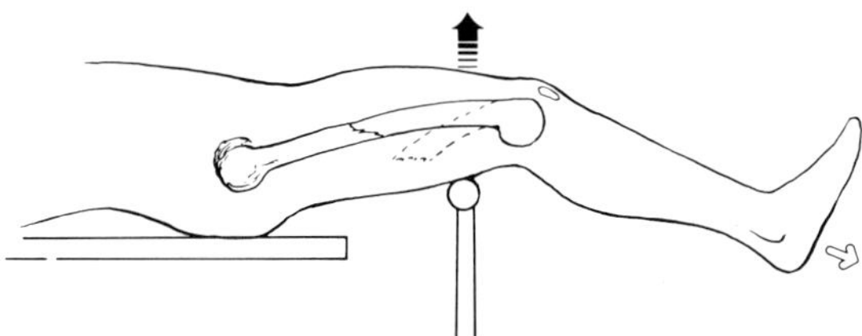

Figure 4–8. The knee rest or countersupport provides an adjustable vertical vector that can be removed more proximally in shaft fractures to affect reduction while the knee is in extension.

Figure 4–6. Rotation of the pin reduces the fracture. The sled runner tip, plus the preshaped pin will allow the passage of the pin across fractures that previously could not be reduced without using the semi-open technique. In passing the fracture, the head of the pin can be rotated and will usually reduce the fracture.

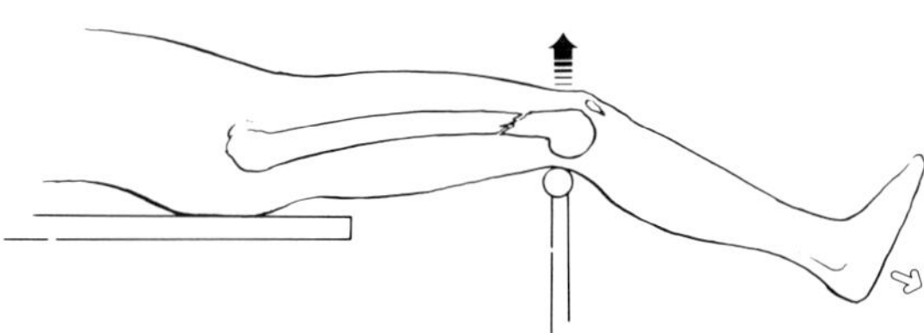

Figure 4–9. The vertical vector or knee rest is moved more distally to resist the pull of the gastrocnemius in supracondylar fractures while the knee is in traction and flexion. These adjustments are all done prior to surgical preparation of the patient.

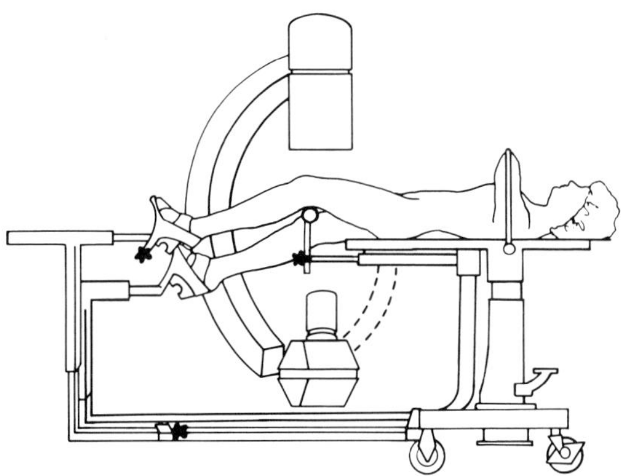

Figure 4–7. Fracture table, developed in 1971 by Dr. Leslie V. Rush, Sr., and manufactured by the Berivon Company, with all important knee rest or countersupport to give a vertical vector force for traction. Extensions to the foot supports are close to the floor allowing the C-arm of the image intensifier to be functional in both the anteroposterior and the lateral view.

at the same time, and surgery can be done simultaneously.

Forcible manipulations of the soft tissues and fractures are usually needed only when internal fixation is delayed. Two simple methods are: The patient is on an extension fracture table, and circumferential manipulation is accompanied by the use of the hands, or the crutch and strap, or the femur wrench, a new sterilizable version of the Thomas wrench (Orthopaedic Systems, Model #5415). With delayed care, forcible manipulation to prove that the fracture is reducible or reduced will make surgery much less difficult.

continual manual traction is not needed. The Berivon Rush table does this well. Were it not for the knee rest or countersupport (Figs. 4–8, 4–9) that can be placed in an appropriate position along the femur to maintain a closed reduction, the Berivon table would be just another fracture table suitable for image intensification. At Orthopaedics-Indianapolis I developed a double knee rest system for use in bilateral femoral fractures so that reduction of both fractures can be obtained

BASIC INSTRUMENTS AND PINS

There are four diameters for the pins (Fig. 4–10): A, ¼ inch (6.35mm) shepherd's crook; B, 3⁄16 inch (4.76mm), regular or 3⁄16 inch (4.76mm), with the looped condylar head; C, ⅛ inch (3.18mm); and D, 3⁄32 inch (2.38mm). Length of pins are labeled

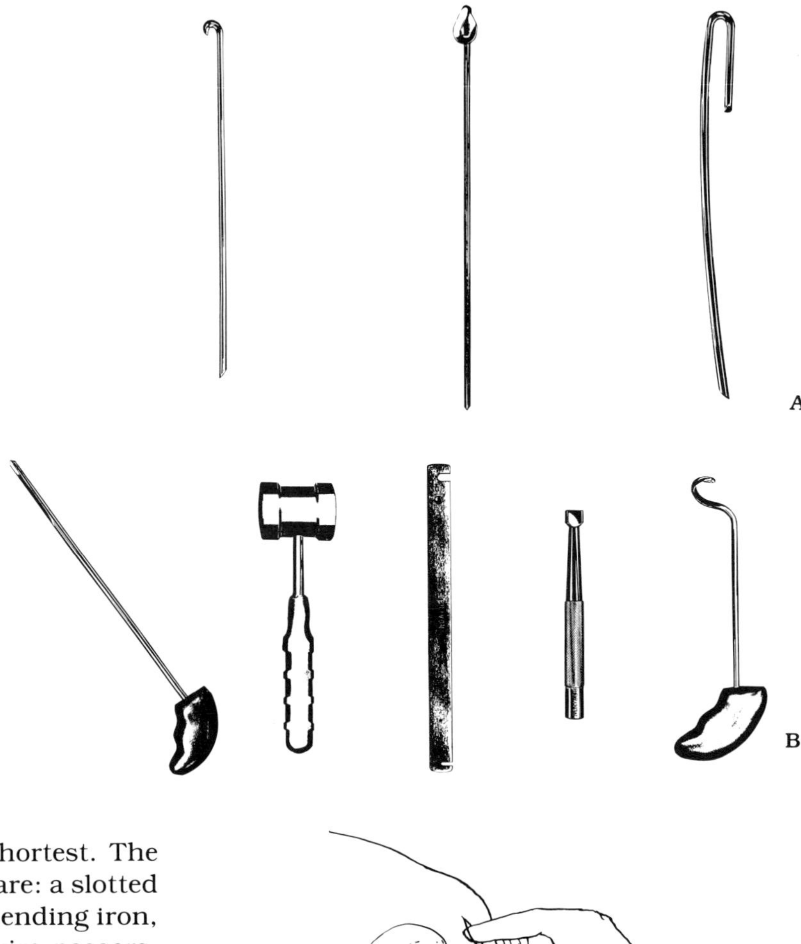

Figure 4–10. (A) Three types of Rush pins (left to right): regular—¼- (6.35mm), ³⁄₁₆- (4.76mm), ⅛- (3.18mm), (2.38mm), ³⁄₃₂-inch diameters; looped condylar— ³⁄₁₆-inch (4.76mm) diameter; and shepherd's crook—¼-inch (6.35mm) diameter. (B) Basic instruments (left to right): awl and impactor—four sizes, mallet, bending iron, and wire passers.

alphabetically, A being the shortest. The instruments (see Fig. 4–10) are: a slotted awl in the four diameters, a bending iron, mallets with a large head, wire passers, impacters in four sizes, and a pin extractor. The knee rest or countersupport separate from the table is also considered a reducing instrument.

SELECTING THE LENGTH OF PIN

The length of pin selected depends on its use (Fig. 4–11). Fixation of diaphyseal fractures depends on pin length to control rotation. Pins that are prebent and static should generally be long. Dynamic pins that develop their curve from intraosseous forces should be much shorter, especially those used in comminuted epiphyseal-metaphyseal fractures, which tend to shorten. In shaft fractures the best way to choose a pin of the proper length is as

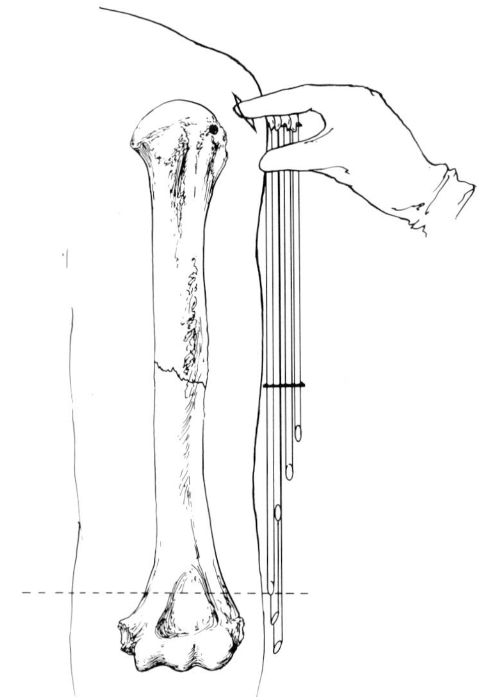

Figure 4–11.   Pin length selection for humerus.

follows: Overcome the shortening of the extremity by traction; choose the rack of pins indicated for the bone, and lay this rack alongside the incision and the awl that is going into the bone; and then measure to the distal end of the extremity.

In epiphyseal-metaphyseal fractures where two pins are used, length is also important. If the pin is too short, continuous forces exerted by the point against the wall of the bone causes the pin to migrate backward, carrying with it the distal fragment, which will result in distraction and nonunion. If the pin is of proper length, lateral pressure is exerted by the shafts of the pins against the wall of the bone. This results in good fixation and permits the shaft of the bone to telescope on the pin so that the muscle pull of the extremity can produce compression of the fractured surfaces to stimulate good healing. When the pin is too long, the pins cross a second time to that the points are impinging forklike against the wall of the bone. Some bone absorption at the fracture site occurs during the healing process. The fracture surfaces may thus be held apart to prevent compression, with the result being delayed healing or nonunion or the pin becoming prominent as the fracture shortens.

Pin insertion techniques are similar for the four pin sizes. Except in young, hard bone, the awl, which has a pointed cutting tip and a cutting slot, is easier to use than a drill. The angle of insertion is the most unforgiving feature of fracture fixation with a Rush pin. Obviously, the sharp point of the awl must penetrate the thin cortical bone at right angles to engage the medullary canal, and then with a scooping motion and use of the slot on the awl to cut the bone and enlarge the hole, the awl is gradually turned to be at a 30-degree angle to the shaft of the bone. For the beginner, this is an excellent time to use the image intensifier to observe and create the proper angle of insertion. This angle is important, for the tip of the pin is beveled and can bounce off the opposite cortex if the awl is inserted properly. If the angle is more than 30 degrees, the tip of the pin may penetrate the opposite cortex and go into the soft tissues.

PRESHAPING THE PIN

Curving the pin with a bending iron is almost routinely done when it is to be used in the shafts of the humerus, femur, and tibia. The convexity of the curve is always away from the point and hook of the head. Determining how much to bend a ¼-inch (6.35mm) pin for stabilization of a shaft fracture of the femur, tibia, or humerus is always difficult. Since rotational control is the reason for preshaping the pin in a shaft fracture, there are two factors that determine the amount: the diameter of the medullary canal at the fracture site and the density of the epiphyseal metaphyseal bone.

Medullary canal size increases with age. Density of the epiphyseal metaphyseal bone decreases with age. Therefore, the amount of curve in a ¼ inch (6.35mm) pin should be more for older people with large canals. A general rule of thumb: The curve produced by the bonding irons should be slightly greater than the diameter of the medullary canal at the fracture site (Fig. 4–12).

Driving the pin is an interesting experience when the impactor is not used. When the pin is pounded down the canal, the head of the pin will rotate as the sled runner tip with its beveled side slides along the medullary canal. Occasionally the tip will get hung up and pliers will be used to untwist it; then the pin continues along the medullary canal. After the pin passes across the fracture site, there will be a change in the sound of impaction, indicating stability of the fracture. With experience, this sound or lack of it deter-

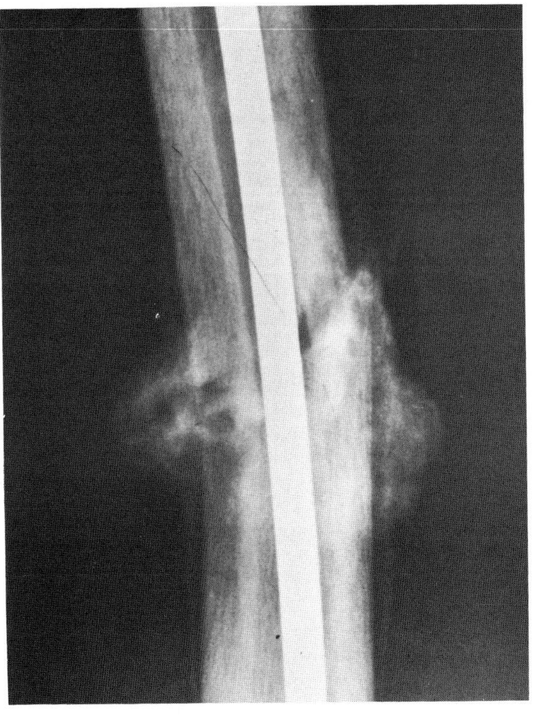
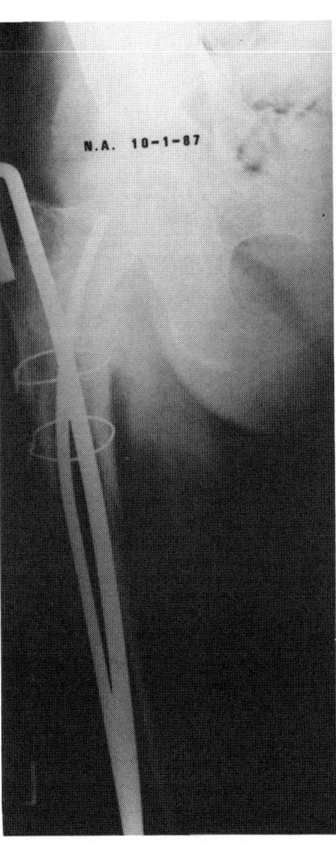

A   B

Figure 4–12.   Medullary canal sizes increase with age. (A) Femur of a 22-year-old man with a narrow medullary canal. It is doubtful whether any additional pin fixation would fit across this narrow canal. (B) An 82-year-old woman who had a spiral subtrochanteric fracture fixed with a shepherd's crook curved Rush pin and a single Ender nail from the medial femoral condyle exhibits the large medullary canal so characteristic of older age groups.

mines whether the surgeon tries again or prepares for seating of the pin. Generally the impactor is needed only for final seating of the head of the pin in the bone. It can also be used to extract the pin. The pliers is one of the best instruments for turning the head of the pin, and thus the sled runner, to facilitate the passage across the fracture site.

Fixation of fractures near joints presents a problem for all fixation devices, but again the soft tissues will help with the stability near the ligamentous and capsular structures. Supracondylar femoral fractures, Colles' fractures and fractures at the ankle are classic examples. Again, the angle of insertion of the awl is critical. The opposite bone (that is, the ulna in the Colles' fracture and the tibia or fibula in the ankle fracture) provides the opposite supporting structure. If both bones are fractured, then an opposing pin is needed, as in the supracondylar fracture of the femur. In short fractures near a joint, the fully inserted pin may tilt the proximal fragment because of its resilient force (Fig. 4–13).

Stress relieving is the term used for bending the pin, already inserted in the bones, near to its head at final insertion in order to decrease the resilient force of the pin. Stress relieving tends to weaken the force of the pin but solves the fixation problem (Fig. 4–14). For Colles' fracture, reduction with a ⅛-inch (3.18mm) pin can angulate the fracture. The pin can be

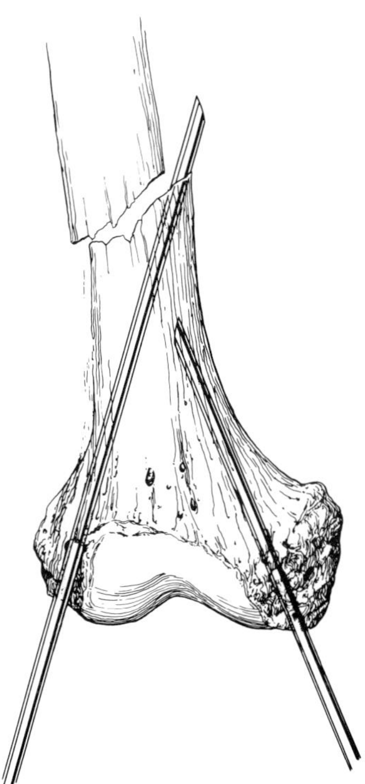

Figure 4–13. Oblique fractures of the femur. When both pins are inserted up to the fracture site, the pin that is in the same obliquity as the fracture must be inserted across the fracture site first by either bending the fracture site to ensure its passage or changing the direction of the pin. After the pin is in the proximal fragment for a short distance, the opposite pin can then be placed across the fracture without difficulty, with heads seated in the bone.

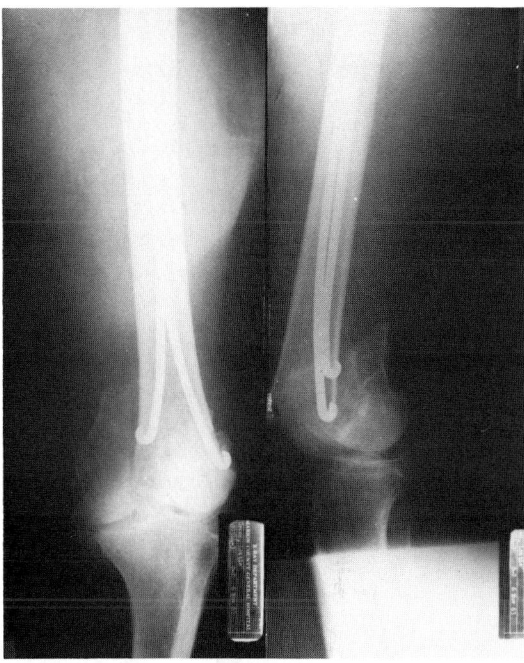

Figure 4–14. Dynamic effects of a resilient pin. If a pin enters obliquely through the side of the bone, it is forced into a curve. Being resilient, it continuously acts to straighten itself and this dynamic force is exerted at three primary points. As a result, if the force is great enough, the head may sink into the bone. More stress relieving of the medial pin or use of a looped condylar pin would have prevented this pin migration into the medullary canal in this supracondylar fracture.

stress relieved to decrease the dynamic force or it can be exchanged for a $\frac{3}{32}$-inch (2.38mm) pin that normally has less force, and this may solve the problem. If the forces are not relieved, the head of the pin may migrate into the medullary canal.

Bending irons are used for three purposes: one, for prebending the pins (Fig. 4–15); two, for stress relieving the pins; and three, for contouring the looped condylar pins for accurate positioning of the loop against soft condylar bone. An excellent article on the pitfalls and safeguards in medullary fixation of fractures with a longitudinal pin was published in the *Mississippi Doctor.*[1]

TUBULATION OF THE BONE BY CERCLAGE WITH WIRE PASSERS

Spiral fractures are low-energy–induced fractures that tend to shorten and rotate. Tubulation by cerclage is the way to prevent this and can provide great stability when used with intramedullary pin fixation. To be used effectively, the wire must be applied without stripping the soft tissue attachments to the bone, for to do so may lessen the healing potential (Fig. 4–16). The soft-tissue attachments keep the wires from sliding into the fracture line or out of position. The tip of the wire passer rubs the periosteum while encircling the

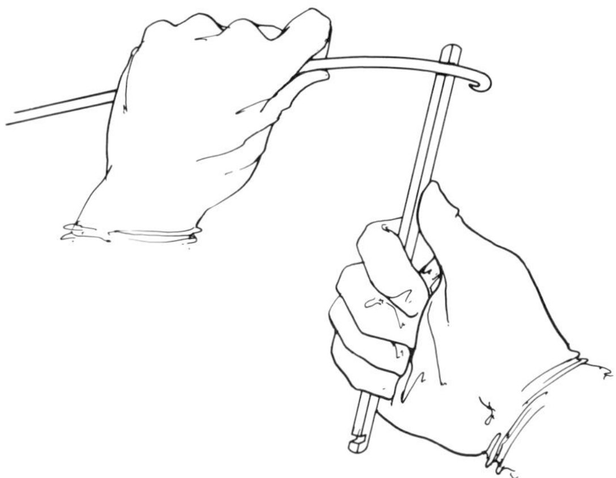

Figure 4–15. Preshaping the pin. Curving the pin with a bending iron is done almost routinely for fixation of shaft fractures of the humerus, femur, and tibia. The convexity of the curve is always away from the point and on the side of the hook of the head. In the forearm, the pin is rarely preshaped. In fractures near joints, the proximal portion of the pin is usually curved with a bending iron just before the pin is driven completely home. This is because a straight pin can be controlled better than a curved one. Only when the proximal portion of the pin needs a curve to conform to the contour of the bone is it best to defer this procedure until the pin has been accurately placed.

bone and avoiding the neurovascular structures. Either No. 18 or No. 16 stainless-steel wire is generally used. The wire is passed about the fracture first, while the fracture is still unstable, and is made ready to tighten. Then the pin is placed in the distal fragment, the cerclage wires are tightened, and the pin is driven home (Fig. 4–17). Any number of wires can be used, the fewer the better. Using one or two is most common. The wire is tightened to the degree that it can just barely be moved with an instrument. A symmetric twist gives the best strength and can be done with wire twisters, pliers, or the jet wire twister.[2]

THE FORMULA FOR OBLIQUE FRACTURES NEAR A JOINT

When a pin is inserted in a short fragment to transfix an oblique fracture near a joint, if possible, the pin should so be directed that the axis of the shaft of the pin tends to parallel the axis of the fracture line. Remember: V for victory and X for no good (Figs. 4–18, 4–19)

DOUBLE PINNING FOR SIMILAR ANATOMIC AREAS

Double pinning is used to provide stability to widened areas of bone, near articular surfaces, and where rotational control of the fracture is difficult to achieve (Fig. 4–20). The pins are usually inserted opposite from each other at the same end of the bone. The most notable exception is fracture in the subtrochanteric region of the femur.

PITFALLS

Backing Out

Pin migration is an early complication but indicates motion at the fracture site. Martens, Frankel, and Burstein[3] stated that the mechanism of pin migration is "repeated angulation in the bending mode"; that is, with angulation of the fracture, the pin bends and shortens slightly, the point catches in the intramedullary cortex, and when the angulatory force reverses, the pin lengthens and protrudes more and more.

Pin Migration into the Medullary Canal

Pin migration occurs when the resiliency of the pin forces it through soft bone to become intramedullary. This is the difficult situation when treating an osteoporotic distal part of the femur or Colles' fracture. Stress relieving of the pin or using the looped condylar pins solves this problem.

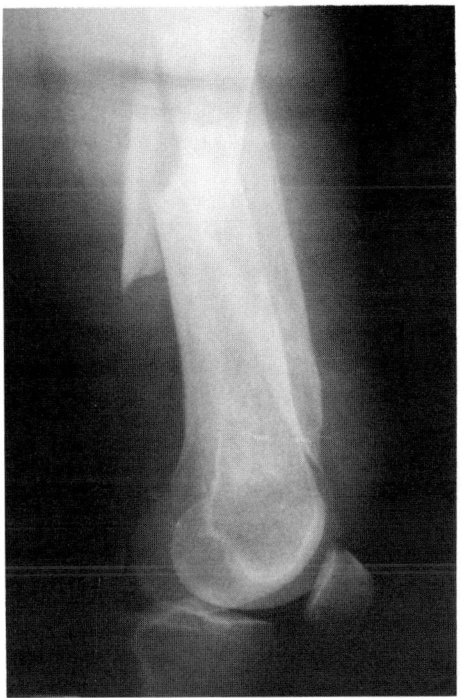

A

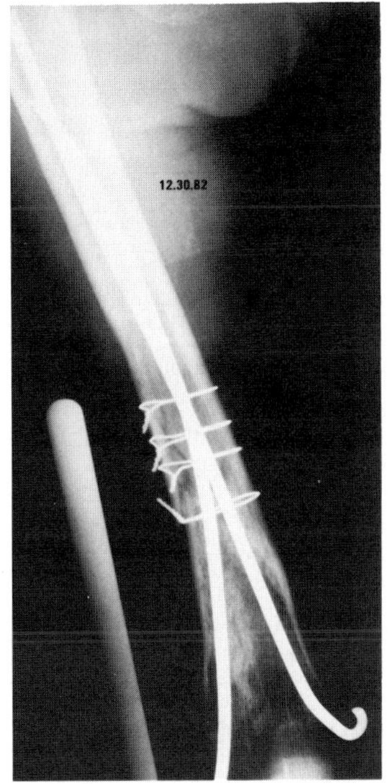

B

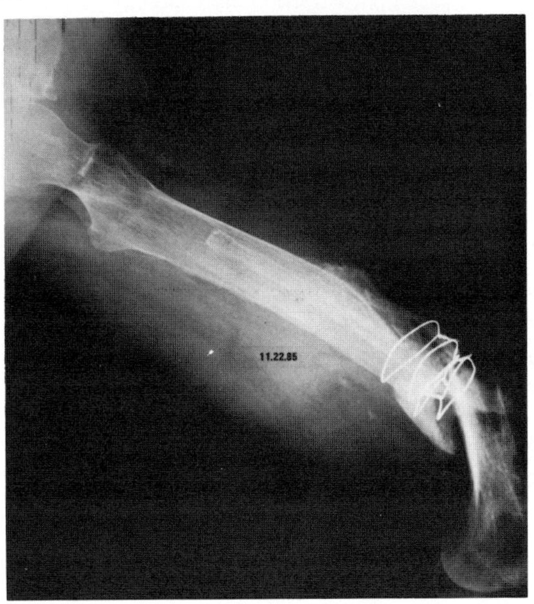

C

Figure 4–16. The effects of excessive cerclage and soft-tissue stripping. (**A**) A 72-year-old female alcoholic had a low-force, spiral, comminuted fracture in the distal part of the femur that turned into a disaster. The disaster was that no healing, external callus occurred. (**B**) The operative note showed extensive stripping for the cerclage wires and pins that were too long and started to re-cross, preventing any shortening. (**C**) The fixation device was removed 3 years later without any attempt to bone graft or internally fix the femur. Using fewer cerclage wires that are tightened less securely and retubulating the bone completely is preferred.

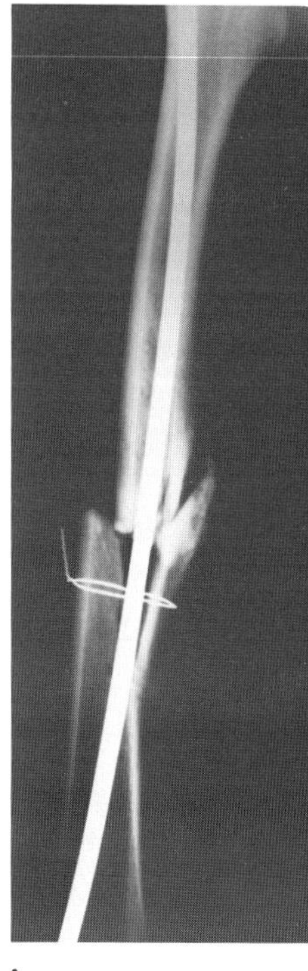

A

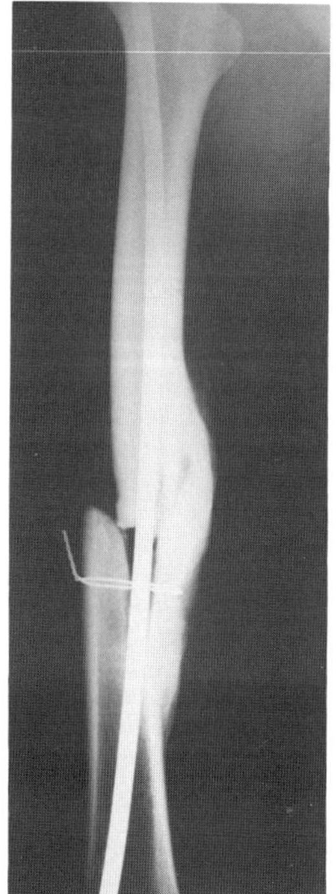

B

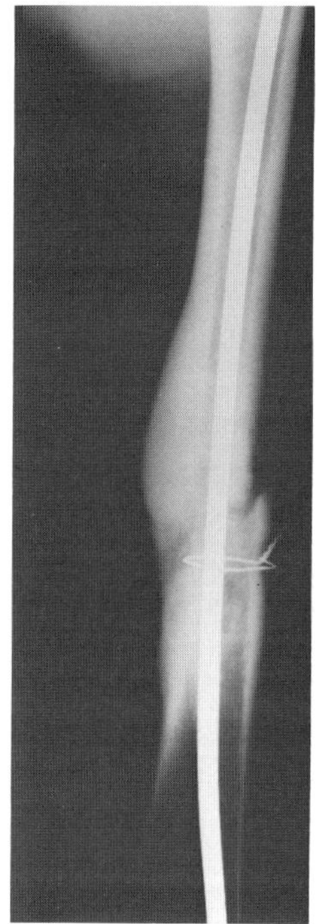

C

Figure 4–17. Retubulation is needed prior to passage of pin. (**A**) The effect is trying to tighten the wire after the pin has been seated in the distal fragment. (**B**) As a result, a fracture wired in June 1979 was partially healed by March 1980. (**C**) By September 1980, it was finally healed.

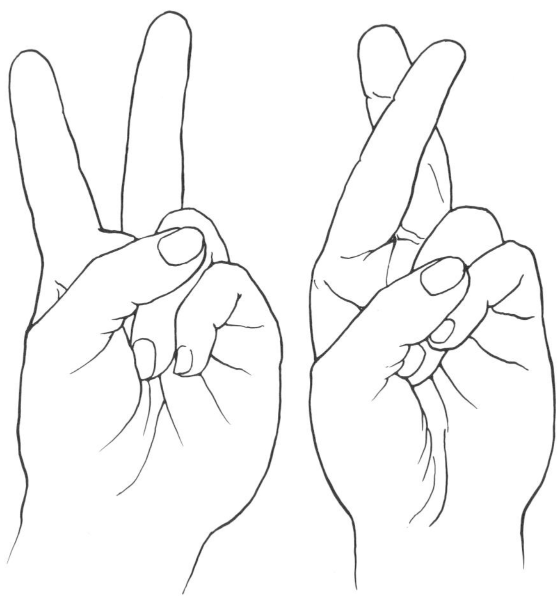

Figure 4–18. *The formula.* V for victory means that the three-point fixation of an oblique fracture near a joint works when the pin runs parallel to the fracture. When the pin forms an X, the three-point pressure forces the fracture apart.

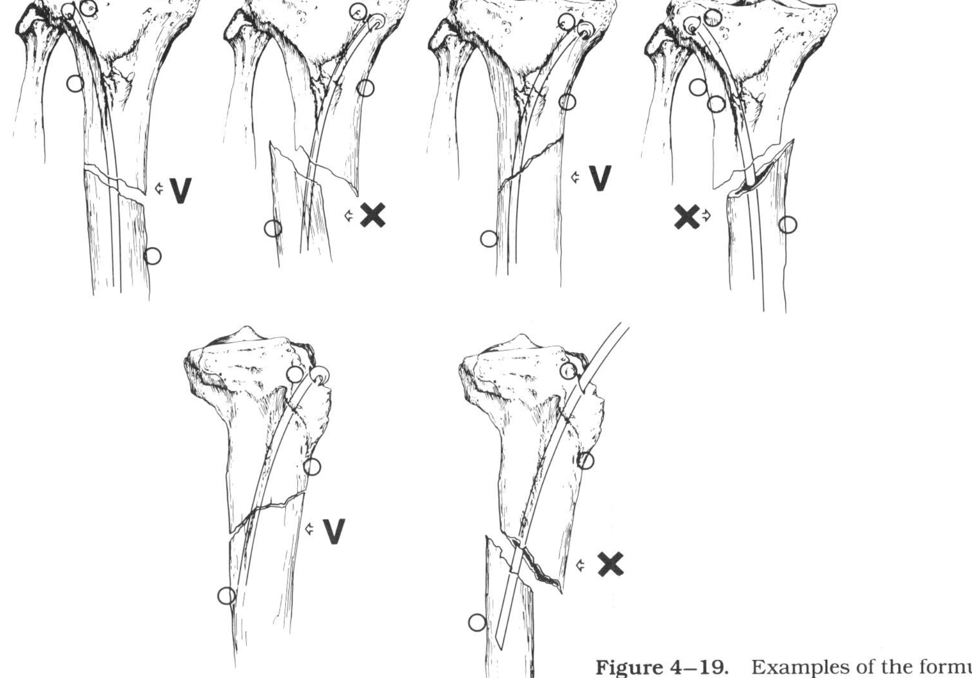

Figure 4–19. Examples of the formula in action.

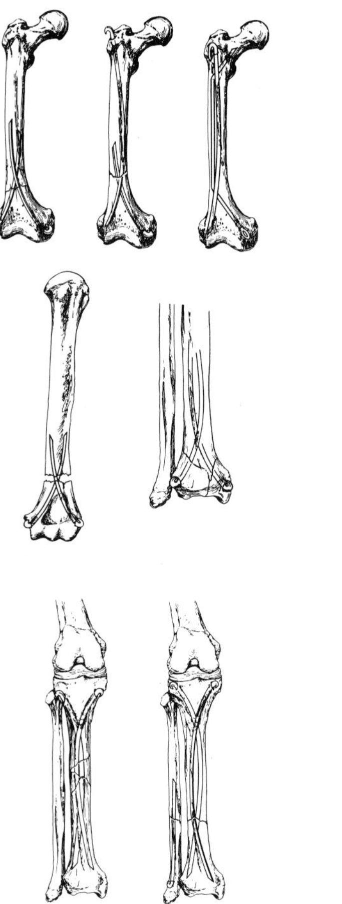

Figure 4–20. Double pinning: similar anatomic areas. The femur, proximal part of the tibia, distal end of the humerus, distal part of the tibia, and proximal subtrochanteric region of the femur.

Metal Failure

Metal failure is almost always the result of the bone failing to heal before the metal fatigues and fails. Slowly healing fractures with minimal callus formation should alert one to nonunion and should be grafted or electrically stimulated early prior to the metal fatigue. Do not rely on the metal. A fatiguing pin should always be exchanged at the time of bone grafting.

REFERENCES

1. Rush, L.V., Rush, H.L.: Pitfalls and safeguards in medullary fixation with the longitudinal pin. Mississippi Doctor January, 378–386, 1950.
2. Quadagni, J.R., Drummond, D.S.: Strength of surgical wire fixation: a laboratory study. Clin. Orthop. 209:176–181, 1986.
3. Martens, M., Frankel, V., Burstein, A.H.: Ultimate properties of intramedullary nails. Injury 4(1):18–24, 1972.

SUGGESTED READINGS

Chapman, M.W.: The role of intramedullary fixation of open fractures. Clin. Orthop. 212:26–34, 1986.
Rush, L.V.: Atlas of Rush Pin Technics. Meridian, Mississippi, The Berivon Company, 1956.
Tscherene, H., Hass, N., Krettek, C.: Intramedullary nailing combined with cerclage wiring in the treatment of fractures of the femoral shaft. Clin. Orthop. 212:62–67, 1986.

Fractures of the Femur

The femur, the bone most frequently surgically treated, is the bone in which the use of prebent or static fixation devices, as well as dynamic one-or two-pin fixation, can be demonstrated (Figs. 5–1, 5–2).

In 1984, a group was formed to study the results of fixation femoral fractures using Rush pins. The group that formed the Indiana Series included the following orthopaedic surgeons: F.R. Brueckmann, D.S. Blackwell, W.O. Irvine, R.A. Hutson, M.R. Stevens, J.C. Randolph, D.E. Russell, T.R. Trammell, A.J. Vicar, V.L. Fragomeni, J.K. Schneider, D.W. Dro, C.C. Reeck, Jr., P.H. Ireland, R.T. Clayton, W.A. Atz, J.G. Crane, D.S. Shelbourne, C.B. Kernek, R.O. Pierce, and D. Heck, all of Indianapolis; T.W. Marshall, R.G. Bennett, and R.L. Forste, Jr., of Columbus, Indiana; R.J. Burkle of Terre Haute, Indiana; R.G. Kleopfer, J.W. Lee, P.A. Reszel, S.R. Glock, A.C. Warr, W.B. LaSalle, J.E. Albright, W.H. Couch, W. Rutledge, and R.G. Caldwell of Fort Wayne, Indiana; J.L. Reynolds of Martinsville, Indiana; R.J. O'Brien of Michigan City, Indiana; S.D. Brandon of DeKalb, Illinois; M.R. Carlson and K.L. Bussey of Champaign, Illinois; M.W. Nelson of Racine, Wisconsin; and D.C. Hadden of Marion, Virginia.

As of November 1987, a total of 785 femurs were treated. There were 701 closed fractures and 66 open or com-

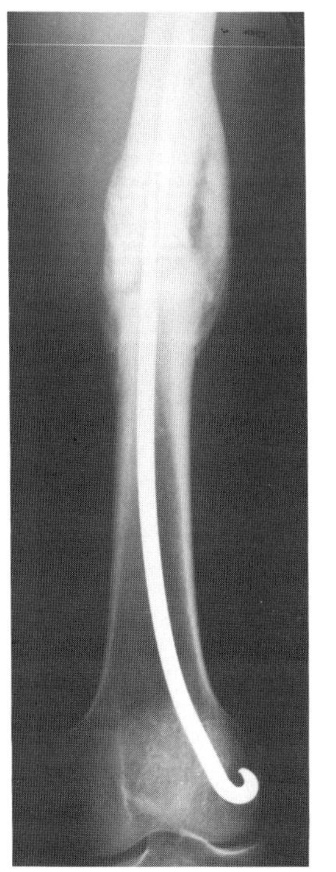
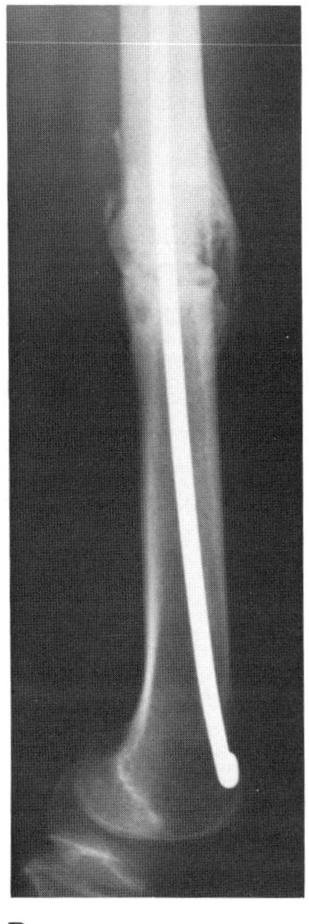
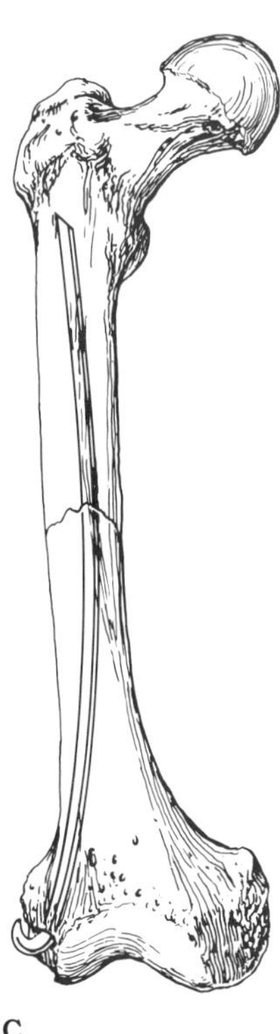

A   B   C

Figure 5–1. Pin fixation from lateral condyle. (**A**) Anteroposterior view. (**B**) Lateral view. (**C**) Prebent ¼-inch (6.35 mm) pin inserted from the lateral femoral condyle.

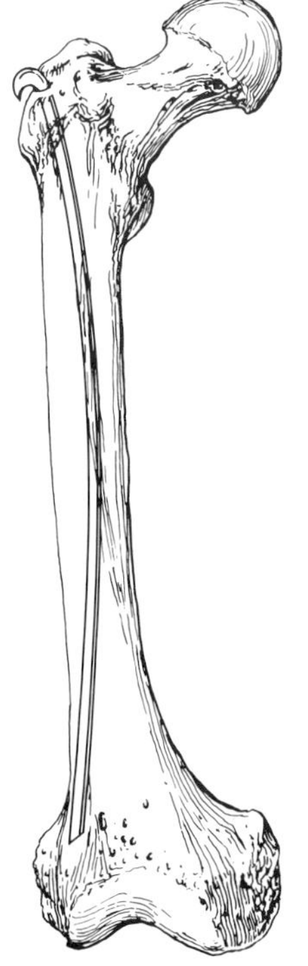

Figure 5–2. Prebent ¼-inch (6.35 mm) pin inserted from the greater trochanter.

pound fractures with 18 pathologic fractures. The distribution was typical, with 34 fractures in the proximal end, 544 shaft fractures, and 208 fractures in the distal end.

These fractures were treated in the manner described by protocol that was distributed at the time as a guideline for treatment. Of the 785 fractures, 625 were treated in a closed fashion after reduction, usually with the patient on the fracture table. In 124 patients fracture treatment was considered as open with either compound or open fractures, semi-open technique treated fractures, or cerclage wire.

Additional implants were seldom used, with 16 screws and 4 Kirschner wires used as supplemental fixation.

Complications were very few, with a total of 23 infections reported, and only 2 established infections at the time of hospital discharge. Eight patients needed a second osteosynthesis during the initial

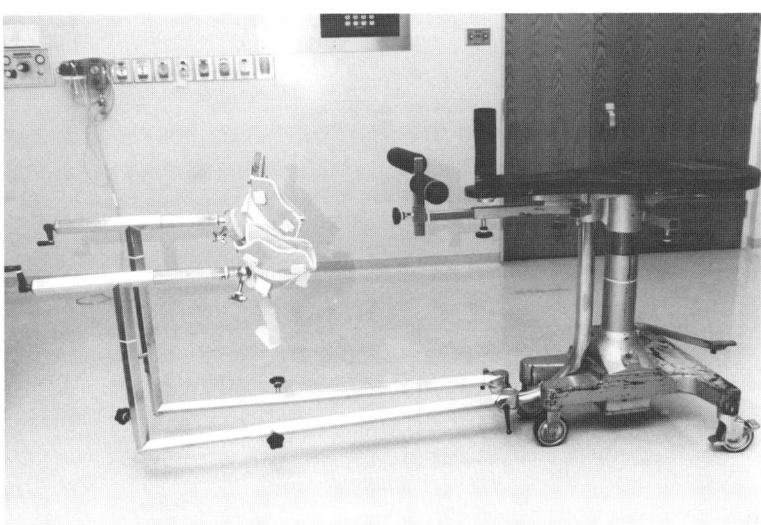

Figure 5–3.   Rush fracture table countersupport for the left femur can be used with image intensifier.

hospitalization, and no metal failures occurred in this group.

At follow-up on 529 patients, 95% followed over 1 to 1½ years, the effects of fixation with a nonreamed pin were striking: 4.1% had nonunion or delayed union; 4.1% had malalignment problems, primarily that of valgus; and 6.0% (32) patients had measurable shortening. These statistics compare almost too favorably with those from other methods and indicate that the method is sound and must be performed technically well by thoughtful surgeons.

Cookbook methods for the use of the basic pin techniques are described in the flow sheet. Single-pin techniques for shaft fractures and two-pin techniques for supracondylar fractures, fractures in the distal one-third and subtrochanteric fractures are shown on the flow sheet. The reduction of the fracture is enhanced by the use of a portable image intensifier. A radiographic knee rest or a countersupport greatly aids in fracture reduction and is essential in the reduction of bilateral fractures of the femoral shaft (Fig. 5–3). The Rush fracture table manufactured by the Berivon Company of Meridian, Mississippi, is the most useful

table available (Fig. 5–4). The closed nailing of a fresh fracture of the femoral shaft with the use of the intensifier best illustrates the technique and is described here and is in the basic pattern for the flow sheet (Fig. 5–5).

Bilateral fractures of the femoral shaft in patients with multiple trauma can be treated simultaneously or at least concurrently in the supine position by using a special bilateral offset knee rest or countersupport devised at Orthopaedics-

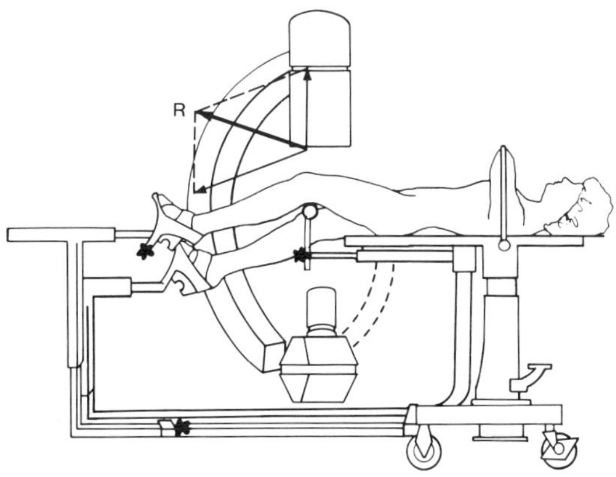

Figure 5–4. Rush fracture table countersupport for the left femur. Note the lowered position of the right femur with legs close together so that anteroposterior and lateral image intensification views can be easily done.

Femoral Fractures Flow Sheet

Step	*Closed Fresh Midshaft, ¼ inch (6.35 mm)*	Single-Pin Technique		
		Closed Delayed Midshaft ¼ inch (6.35 mm)	*Semi-Open Technique ¼ inch (6.35 mm)*	*Closed Spiral or Comminuted Shaft ¼ inch (6.35 mm)*
1. Necessary instruments				
2. Anesthetize patient on table				
3. Put both legs in traction, lower foot				
4. Adjust knee rest				
5. Manipulate & image		Easy Difficult		
6. Difficult reduction	Easy reduction			
7. Prepare skin & drape				
8. Incision			2 incisions	2 incisions
9. Awl technique				Wire passer
10. Awl technique			Manipulate fracture with fingers	Awl
11. Measure length				
12. Bend pin				
13. Check awl position				
14. Exchange pin for awl				
15. Turn sled runner around				
16. Drive in pin to fracture				
17–20. Pin to manipulate fracture				
21. Drive pin in				
22. Impact & inspect				
23. Check radiographs				
24. Close wounds				
25–26. Anterior splint at 90 degrees				

The flow sheet demonstrates methods of treatment for femur fractures. For example, the closed fresh midshaft transverse fracture is shown in a step by step fashion. The flow sheet also lists both single and double pin techniques, as well as static and dynamic fixation.

Two-Pin Technique				
Supracondylar 3/16 inch (4.76 mm)	*Supracondylar T or Y 3/16 inch (4.76 mm)*	*Comminuted Supracondylar 3/16 inch (4.76 mm)*	*Subtrochanteric 6.35 mm + Enders*	*Closed Distal Middle One-third 6.35 mm + 4.76 mm*
			Special 1/4-inch (6.35 mm) pin & Ender pins	Regular 1/4-inch (6.35 mm) & 3/16-inch (4.76 mm) Rush pins
Difficult reduction		Difficult Reduction		
2 incisions		3 incisions	2 incisions—greater trochanter and medial femoral condyle	2 incisions-greater trochanter, medial femoral condyle
	1/8-inch 3.18 mm awl across reduced condyle		1/4-inch (6.35 mm) awl into top of greater trochanter	
Awl technique lateral—judge hardness of bone			Ender awl near adductor tubercle	
Awl technique medial				
			Bend gentle curve 1/4-inch (6.35 mm)	
Check awl position		Cerclage wire		
Exchange pin for awl				
			Measure Ender pin	
Insert pin which is in same plane as oblique fracture first			Insert special pin first	
Alternately unpact			Insert Ender pin	
Stress relieve when 3 to 4 inches remaining			Loosen, impact, image	3/16-inch (4.76 mm) Rush pin
Impact pins, head under capsule			Closure	Image
				Closure

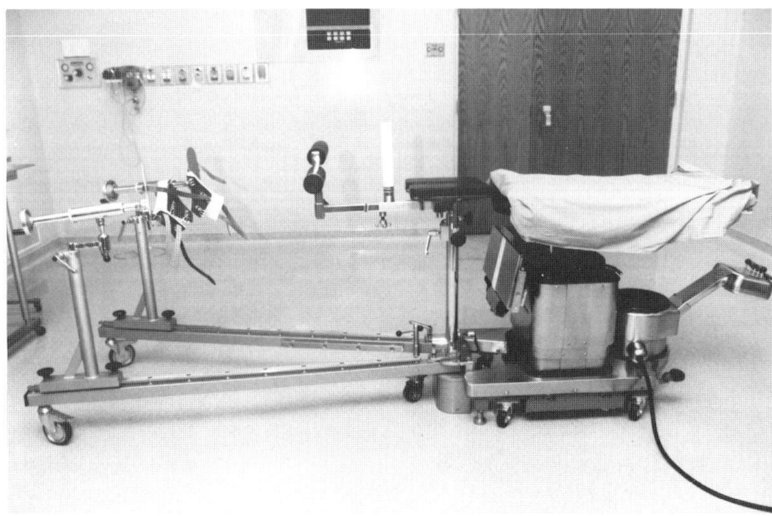

Figure 5–5. Modified Maquet extension table position for the knee countersupport, added to regular operating table.

Indianapolis. The countersupports are at different levels so that on the lateral radiograph, one can discern which femur is actively being treated at the time, even though the two femurs are superimposed. The legs are held parallel to each other, which makes the anterioposterior radiograph easy to obtain.

SINGLE PIN TECHNIQUE

Closed Pinning of Fresh Midshaft Fractures of the Femur with Use of the Image Intensifier

1. Have all the necessary Rush instruments and proper surgical implants of ³⁄₁₆-inch (4.76 mm) and ¼-inch (6.35 mm) diameters available. (Refer to Flow Sheet on page 28.)
2. Place the anesthetized patient on the Rush fracture table with the knee rest on the fractured side and fasten both feet to the foot plates.
3. Lower the foot of the nonfractured side so that the hip is in slight extension with longitudinal traction.
4. Place the knee rest under the knee of the affected femur so that both the hip and the knee are in slight flexion.
5. Manipulate the fractured extremity, using appropriate traction and direct pressure, under image intensification, to evaluate the potential for closed alignment of the fracture (Fig. 5–6).
6. If the fracture is difficult to reduce, plan to introduce the pin from the greater trochanter. This will allow easier reduction when the pin tip is at the fracture site due to improved control of the proximal segment by manipulation of the pin that still extends from the hip.
7. Prepare the skin from the iliac crest to the knee and appropriately drape.

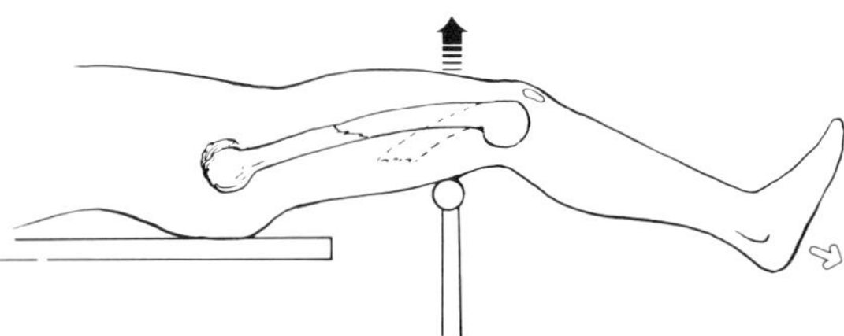

Figure 5–6. Countersupport adjusted with leg in traction to reduce the posterior bowing of the fracture.

8. Use a midlateral incision overlying the greater trochanter. Split the fascia lata and palpate the lateral portion of the greater trochanter at the origin of the vastus lateralis midway between its anterior and posterior borders.

9. Start the ¼-inch (6.35 mm) awl at right angle to the shaft.

10. (A) If introduction of the awl is difficult or if the proximal fragment externally rotates, a bone clamp such as the Bishop clamp should be used to control the proximal fragment while inserting the awl. (b) Use a scooping motion with the sharp edge of the slot of the awl, cutting into the trochanter and gradually changing the angle from 90 degrees to 30 degrees to the long axis of the shaft of the femur. Do not insert the awl past its cutting surfaces.

11. With the awl in the femur, measure the distance from the awl hole to the proximal pole of the patella using a rack of ¼-inch (6.35 mm) Rush pins. The image intensifier is helpful to demonstrate that the pin will reach the femoral condyle.

12. Preshape the pin into a gentle bend using a bending iron. Young patients with small medullary canals require less of a bend than elderly patients with wide medullary canals. Use the image intensifier with the pin overlying the thigh to determine whether the curve is sufficient. The curve will usually effectively shorten the pin about ½ inch, and the tip should end up at the level of the midfemoral condyle when curved (Fig. 5–7).

13. Check the 30-degree angle of the awl insertion with the image.

14. Exchange the ¼-inch (6.35 mm) pin for the awl by sliding the sled runner tip in the slot of the awl.

15. Turn the head of the pin so that the sled runner on the opposite end will face the medial aspect of the medullary canal.

16. Directly impact the pin with the mallet. The use of the impactor may cause difficulty, as the pin normally twists during advancement, and this would be prevented if the impactor held the head of the pin firmly. Failure to note this twisting as the pin advances implies an extramedullary location of the pin.

17. When the pin is at the fracture site, as seen on the image: (A) If the fracture is reduced, drive the pin across. (B) If the fracture is not reduced, manipulate the fracture (Fig. 5–8) using either the pin in the proximal part or manipulate the distal fragment so that the canals are opposed.

18. Drive the pin across the fracture. The sound of impaction will change as stability increases.

19. If the pin misses the distal fragment by sliding over the cortex, use pliers and twist the pin and the sled runner

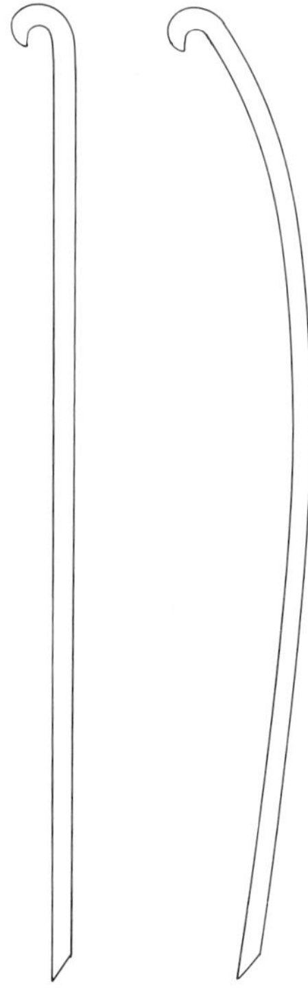

Figure 5–7. One-fourth-inch pins are manufactured straight and must be prebent to fit the medullary canal diameter.

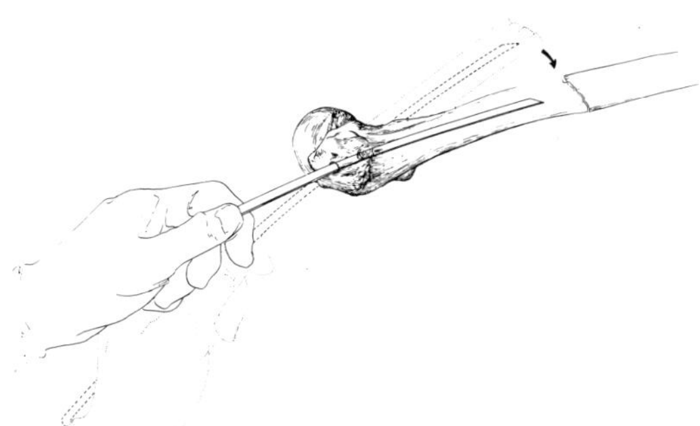

Figure 5–8. Single-pin technique for insertion of the pin at the greater trochanteric area. After the pin has been moved down the shaft, then the pin can be used to manipulate the femur if reduction is not perfect.

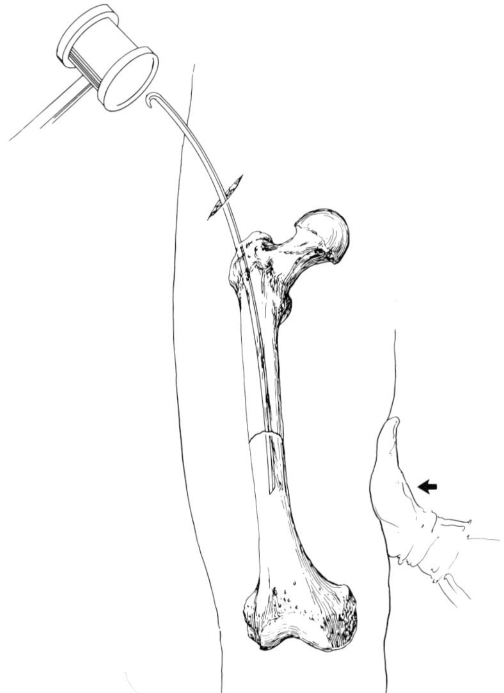

Figure 5–9. After the pin is impacted across the fracture, pressure at the fracture site is used to direct the curved pin into the lateral femoral condyle and give rotational control.

so the tip will slide into the medullary canal. Impact the pin across the fracture, then twist the head back to its original position.

20. If the closed reduction attempts be-

come impossible or impractical, use the semi-open technique and make an incision anterolaterally at the fracture site large enough to admit at least two fingers and manipulate the fracture as described in Nos. 17, 18, and 19.

21. After the ¼-inch (6.35 mm) pin has entered the distal fragment, angulate the fracture into varus position such that the impacted pin tip will be directed into the lateral femoral condyle (Fig. 5–10).

22. With the impactor in place and continued pressure toward a varus angulation, impact the pin into the femoral condyle and seat the hook in the greater trochanter.

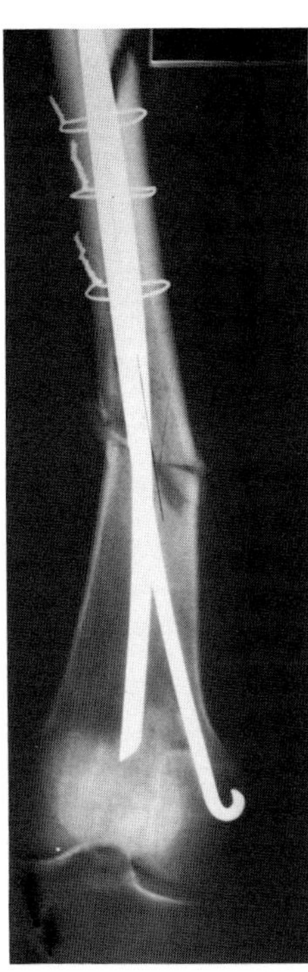

Figure 5–10. In this comminuted segmental fracture, an attempt should have been made to place the tip of the ¼-inch (6.35 mm) pin into the lateral femoral condyle by varus stressing of the femur as the tip entered the distal fragment, though the pin ended up in the middle of the femur. Then the ³⁄₁₆-inch (4.76 mm) pin was inserted across the fracture site and ensured the valgus position of the fracture.

23. Check the anteroposterior and lateral views on the image intensifier.
24. Close the incisions in the usual manner.
25. If this is the only fracture, hold the knee in an anterior plaster splint with the leg at right angles so that the leg can be elevated postoperatively.
26. Postoperatively after the soft tissues have become comfortable, the patient can be set up in bed, the splint removed with the leg hanging again at right angles, and active knee extension can be started (Figs. 5–11, 5–12, 5–13).

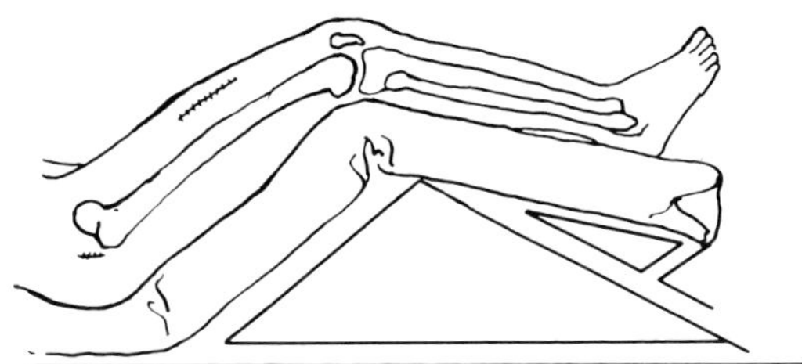

Figure 5–12. Postoperative position in bed, with the hip and knee flexed in the Gatch position.

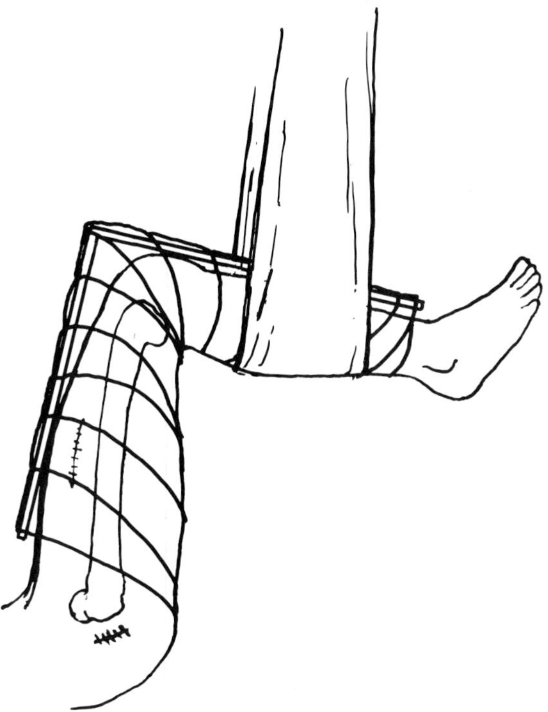

Figure 5–11. A single femoral fracture. Postoperative fixation with an anterior cast held with an Ace bandage and suspended to the overhead frame will in a few days allow sufficient comfort so that the patient can sit up with the leg dependent, the cast can be removed, and knee extension exercises initiated from a right angle.

Closed Pinning of Delayed Midshaft Fractures Using Image Intensifier

1. Have the necessary instruments and implants of ¼-inch (6.35 mm) diameter available.
2. Place the anesthetized patient on the fracture table with the knee rest on the fractured side and fix both feet to the appropriate foot plates.
3. Lower the foot of the nonfractured side so that the hip is in slight extension and put longitudinal traction on it.
4. Place the knee rest under the knee of the affected femur so that the hip and the knee are in slight flexion.
5. Manipulate in traction by using the crutch and strap technique or a knee wrench to loosen the fracture while viewing with the image intensifier (Fig. 5–14). Continued traction may actually completely reduce it at this time. If it is reduced at this time and will stay reduced, return to No. 6 of the technique of closed pinning of the femur and continue to No. 26.
6. If an easy reduction of the fracture is possible, then insertion of the pin from the lateral femoral condyle is the easiest method.
7. Prepare the skin surgically from the iliac crest to the knee and drape appropriately.

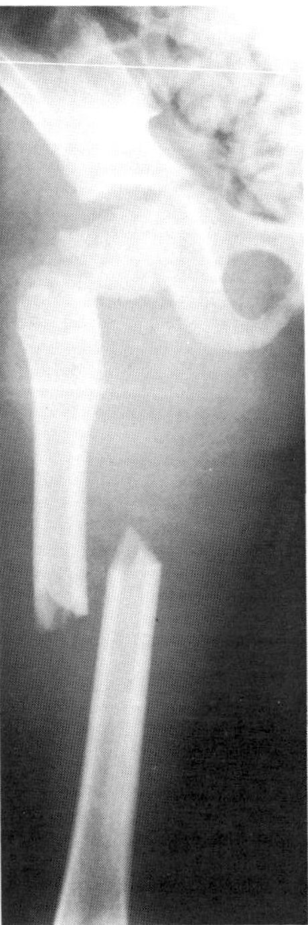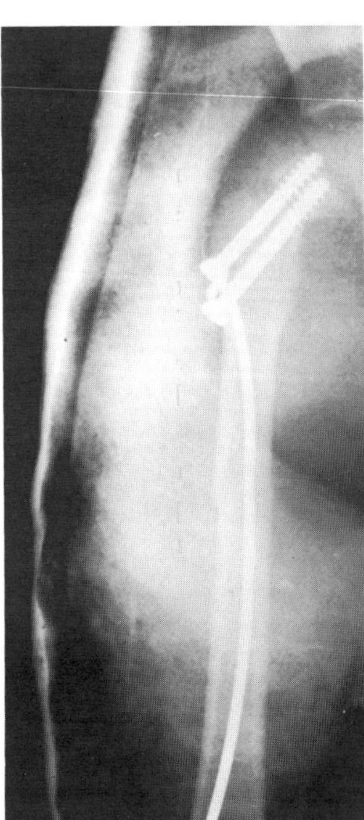

A   B

Figure 5–13. Spica cast can be used in children. (**A**) A 7-year-old girl with a combination femoral neck and shaft fracture and head injury. At the time of delayed surgery, traction was placed on the femur and the femoral neck fracture reduced. Surgically, the greater trochanter was visualized. (**B**) Cannulated screws were placed across the neck fracture. After stabilization of the neck fracture, a ³⁄₁₆-inch (4.76 mm) awl was inserted between the screw heads and a precurved ³⁄₁₆-inch (4.76 mm) pin was passed across the irregular shaft fracture, closed, and provided stable fixation. A spica cast was added as security

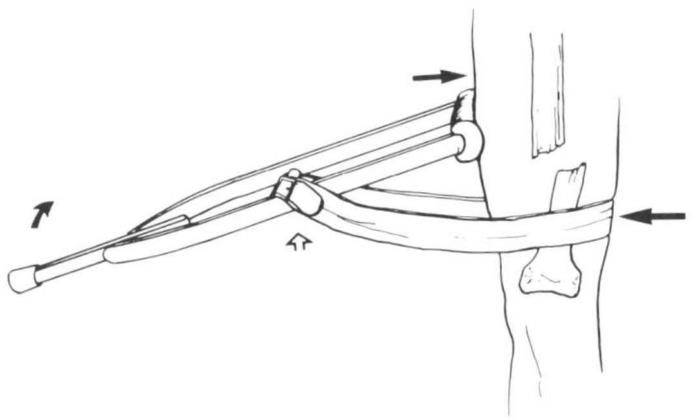

Figure 5–14.   Manipulation by crutch and strap.

8. Make a lateral knee incision at the midcondyle in line with the femoral shaft about ¾-inch (2 cm) posterior to the articular surface so that the joint is entered.

9. Insert the awl into the femur at the superior part of the incision at right angles; try to assess how hard the bone is to penetrate at this time.

10–23. Refer to the Flow Sheet on page 28 for the single-pin technique of closed pinning of femoral midshaft fractures.

24. Close the lateral knee incision after the head of the pin is inserted and seated, so that the head of the pin is underneath the capsule in the fascia lata.

25, 26. Refer to Flow Sheet on page 28 for the single-pin closed pinning of fresh fractures of the femoral shaft.

Semi-Open Technique for Closed Pinning of Femoral Midshaft Fractures without Radiographic Control

1–4. Refer to Flow Sheet on page 28.

5. Manipulate the femur and attempt to get length using traction with the fracture table, and feel the fracture move.

6–7. Refer to Flow Sheet on page 28.

8. Make an anterolateral incision at the level of the fracture site through the fascia, split the vastus lateralis, and palpate the fracture site with a finger.

9. Insert the awl either at the level of the greater trochanter or at the lateral femoral condyle after proper surgical approach and then gradually change the angle of the awl to 30 degrees, aiming toward the palpable fracture site (Fig. 5–15).

10. Manipulate the fracture with the fingers.

11, 12. Refer to Flow Sheet on page 28.

13. When the awl has been directed to a 30-degree angle to the long axis of the femur, it should be pointing in the same plane as the femur, with the fingers at the fracture site.

14–16. Refer to Flow Sheet on page 28.

17. When the ¼-inch (6.35 mm) pin exits the proximal fragment, back the pin up and reduce the fracture by direct manipulation, and if it is not reducible, go to No. 17(b) of the single-pin technique for closed pinning of fresh femoral shaft fractures (Fig. 5–16).

18–22. Refer to Flow Sheet on page 28 (Fig. 5–17).

23. Obtain anteroposterior and lateral radiographs.

24–26. Refer to Flow Sheet on page 28.

Spiral or Large-Piece Comminuted Fractures of the Femoral Shaft

1. In addition to the usual ¼-inch (6.35 mm) Rush pins and instru-

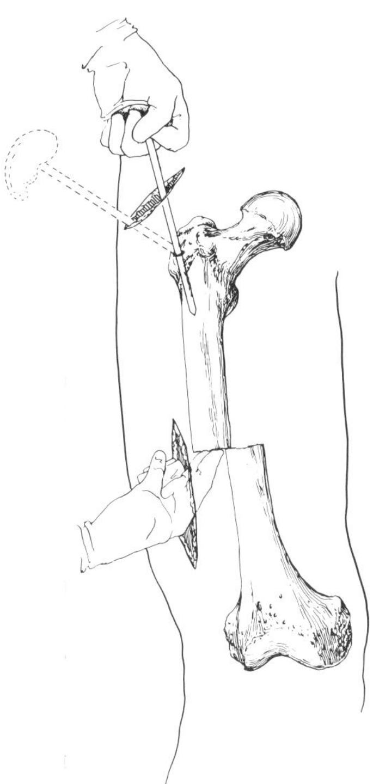

Figure 5–15. The semi-open technique for shaft fractures, with the palpating finger touching the shaft fracture while the awl is directed appropriately at the greater trochanter.

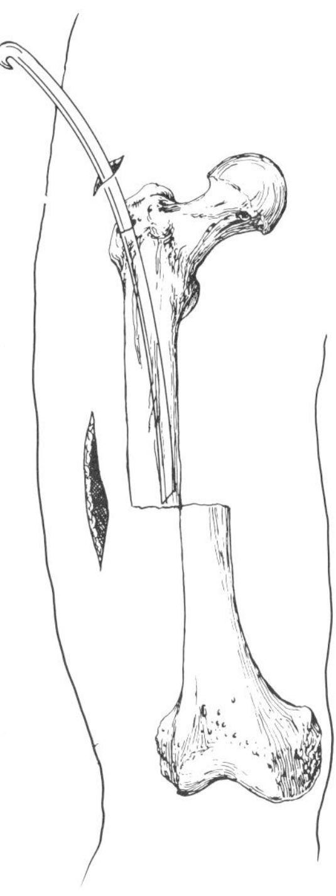

Figure 5–16. If the pin goes out of the fracture, the pin is backed out. The finger is used to reduce the fracture or the pin can be twisted to allow the sled runner to cross the fracture and reduce it.

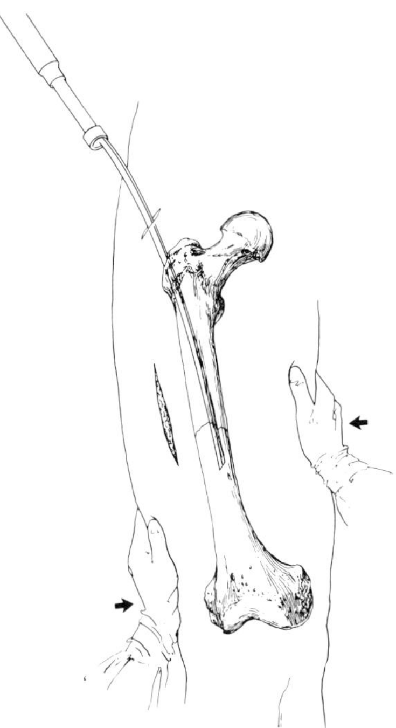

Figure 5–17.   The pin is placed across the fracture site and then a varus deformity is produced by manipulation, and the curved pin is impacted to enter the lateral femoral condyle.

ments, have a wire passer and No. 16 and 18 stainless-steel malleable wire available (Fig. 5–18). Use the technique described for single-pin semi-open technique.

2–8. Refer to Flow Sheet on page 28.

9. Make an anterolateral incision at the fracture site. Do minimal additional dissection and use a wire passer, passing the wire without stripping the muscle from the bone. Usually two or three wires are sufficient, and the wire should be tightened sufficiently so that one can barely move the wire on the bone when the wire is tight (Fig. 5–19).

10–16. Refer to Flow Sheet on page 28.

17. When the pin is at the fracture as seen on the image intensifier: (A) If the fracture is reduced, pound the pin across the fracture. (B) If the fracture is not reduced, ma-

nipulate the fracture by using the pin in the proximal part of the femur or manipulate the distal part of the femur into a reduction. (C) When the pin is at the fracture site, if it tries to come out of the spiral fracture line, twist the head of the pin to change the direction of the sled runner tip before inserting the pin across into the opposite fragment.

18. Impact the pin across the fracture.

19. If the pin misses the distal fragment by sliding over the cortex, use pliers and twist the sled runner so that it will slide into the medullary canal. After it goes across the fracture, then retwist the head back to its previous position.

20, 21. After the ¼-inch (6.35 mm) pin has entered the distal fragment, attempt to hold the fracture in some varus position by pressing medially at the fracture site and laterally at the knee, and this will attempt to direct the pin into the lateral femoral condyle.

22. When the impactor is in place and pressure is toward a varus position, impact the pin into the femoral condyle and seat the hook into the greater trochanter.

23. Check anteroposterior and lateral views on the image intensifier.

24. Close the incisions in the usual manner.

25. If this is the only fracture, hold the knee in an anterior plaster splint with the leg at right angles so that the leg can be elevated postoperatively.

26. After the soft tissues become comfortable, the patient may sit up in bed, the splint can be removed, and with the leg hanging at right angles, active knee extension can be started (Fig. 5–20).

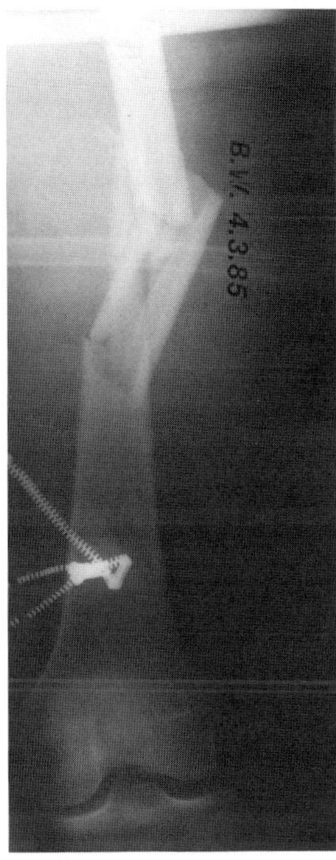
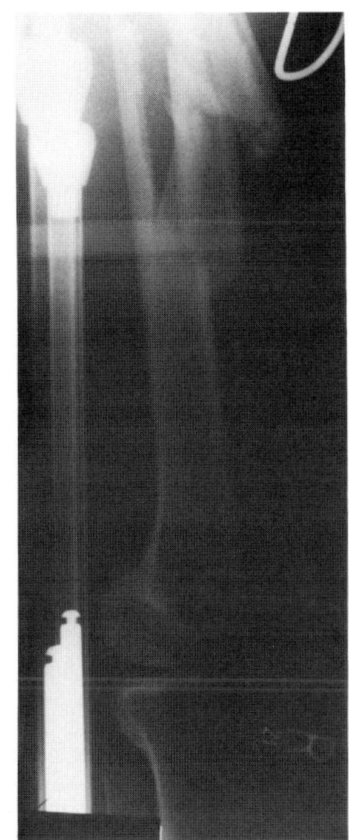

A

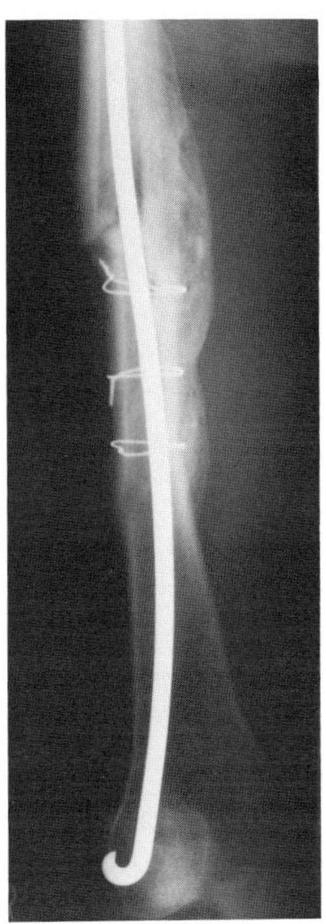
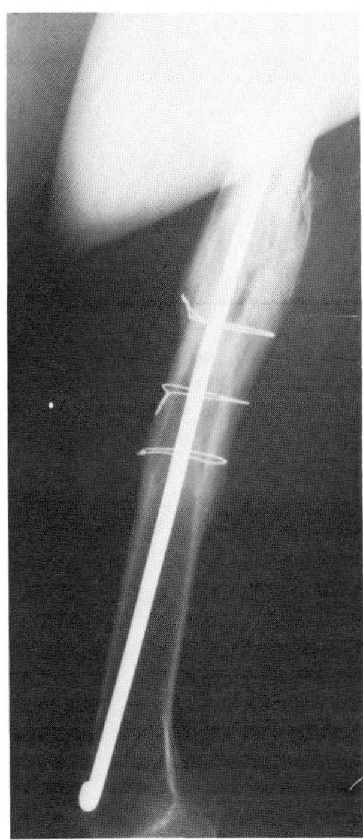

B

Figure 5–18. Comminuted femoral shaft fracture. (**A**) A 32-year-old motorcylist had fracture of both bones in the forearm, plus a comminuted femoral shaft fracture. The femoral fracture was reduced on the fracture table incompletely. A precurved ¼-inch (6.35 mm) pin was started in the lateral femoral condyle. A 5 inch (10 cm) lateral anterolateral incision was placed in the area of the comminuted fractures and two cerclage wires were passed with minimal stripping of muscles. By twisting the head of the precurved pin, the sled runner tip passed into the proximal fragment, and the head was re-twisted so that the pin could be inserted into the greater trochanter. Surgical time was 40 minutes. A third cerclage wire was passed and the wounds closed. The patient was not able to walk because of his forearm fracture. (**B**) Radiographs at 3 months show a healed femur with painless weight-bearing.

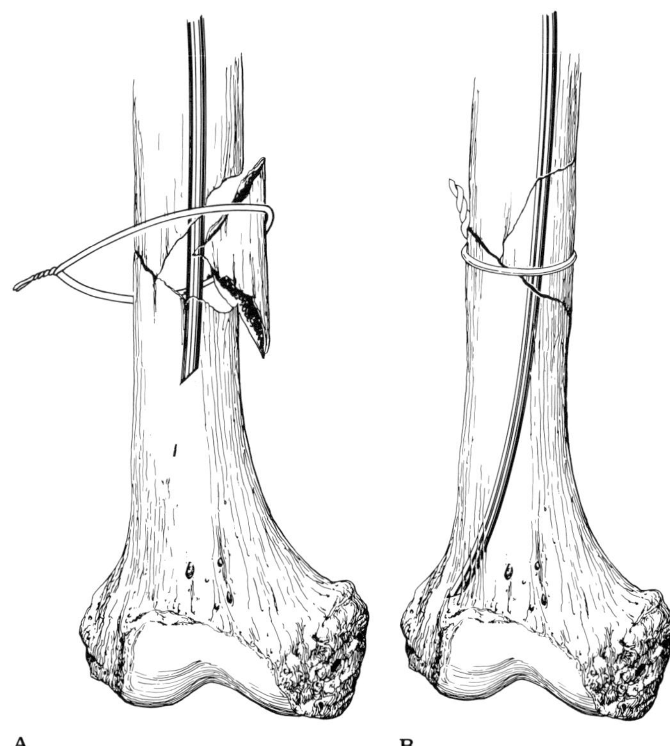

Figure 5–19. (**A**) Cerclage wire is passed with wire passer close to the bone and tightened prior to or while the pin is just across the fracture site. (**B**) After the wire is tightened, the precurved pin is seated in the lateral femoral condyle.

A

B

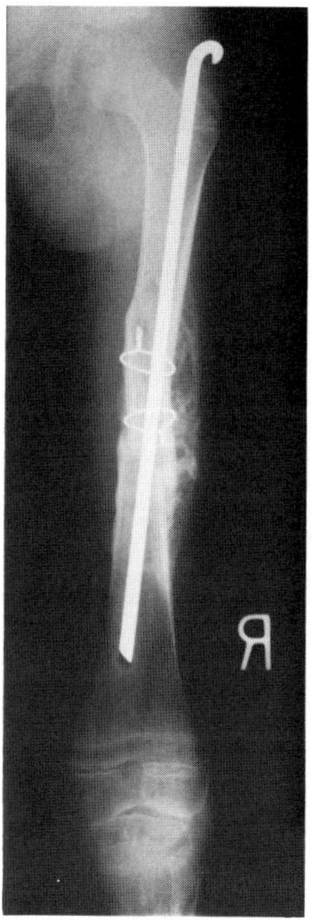
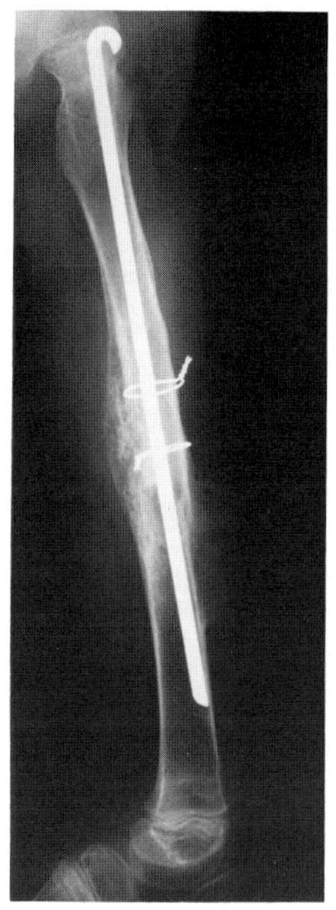

Figure 5–20. A 4-year-old girl with severe brain damage, almost continuous convulsions, and a ruptured spleen, had a split segmental fracture with 2½-inches of femur lying transverse to the shaft. Attempts at closed reduction were impossible. A pin was inserted medial to the proximal trochanteric apophysis and an anterolateral incision revealed the longitudinally split segmental fracture to be completely devoid of all muscle. The fracture was wired together on the operating stand and shish-kabobed, and then the pin advanced distally to miss the distal femoral epiphysis. The head of the pin was left more proximal than the greater trochanter, and a hip spica cast was applied. The pin and spica were removed at 3 months, with fracture healing.

Single-pin techniques for fixation of shaft fractures using the semi-open technique and those with comminution are quite similar because the fracture site is opened to reduce the fracture manually and to pass a cerclage wire. Again, the prebending of the ¼-inch (6.35 mm) pin and the sled runner tip greatly enhance reduction as the tip of the pin will be able to search out the opposite medullary canal and then go into the medullary canal, and with further impaction reduce the fracture with comminution and large enough fragments. A wire passer and No. 16 or 18 stainless-steel wire should be used without stripping the muscle from the bone. The tip should hug the femur and, especially while going through the tough linea aspera, the passage may be difficult. In tightening a cerclage wire, traction at the same time of twisting is necessary to make a strong twist and not to break the wire.

TWO-PIN TECHNIQUES

Dynamic Two-Pin Fixation of Supracondylar Femoral Fractures

The most impressive location for fixation using two ³⁄₁₆-inch (4.76 mm) Rush pins, either regular or the looped condylar pin for soft bone, is the supracondylar area. The straight resilient pins, when deflected from the opposite cortex, are forced into a curve which dynamically compresses the heads of the pins toward each other. This is helpful to compress the split in T or Y fractures. It may be harmful if the bone is soft, as the pins may cut into the medullary canal. Soft bone, as determined on insertion of the awl, should indicate the use of loop condylar pins or stress relieving of the pins. Several points previously mentioned are repeated here (Fig. 5–21):

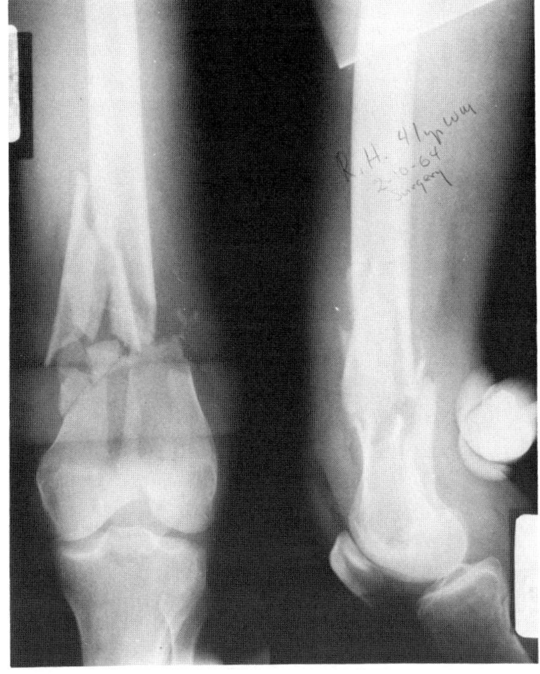

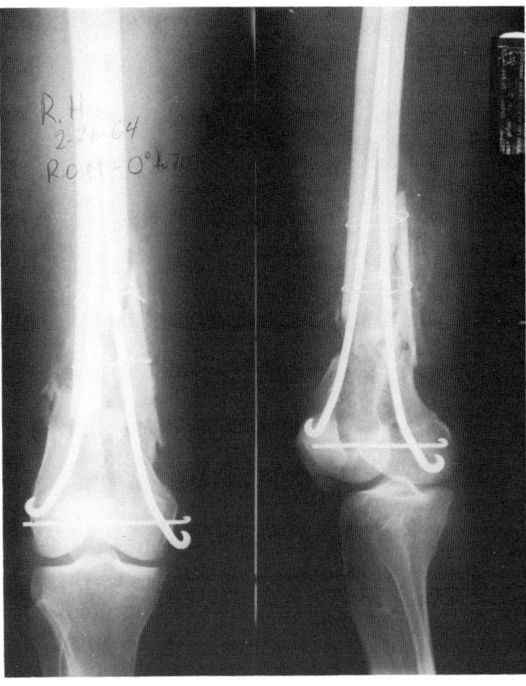

A   B

Figure 5–21.   Rapid healing of comminuted supracondyla fracture. () A 41-year-old man with intracondylar and comminuted supracondylar fracture who was treated on regular fracture table and table countersupport with two ³⁄₁₆"inch (4.76 mm) pins, cerclage wires, and a ³⁄₃₂-inch (2.38 mm) transverse pin. (**B**) Note the callus formation in 16 days and the compression of the condyles, making the transverse pin too long.

1. The pins should be driven simultaneously to prevent displacing the shaft.
2. Pins should not be too long. They can impinge and give distraction and nonunion. With comminution the fractures may shorten and the pins remain, thus becoming protuberant underneath the capsule and skin.
3. Pins that are too short will migrate backward.
4. For oblique fractures of the proximal supracondylar area, the pin that would normally go out the fracture should be placed in first or it will be impossible to reduce the fracture and pin it.

Supracondylar Fractures of the Femur

1. Have all the proper instruments available including ³⁄₁₆-inch (4.76 mm) awl, impactors, bending irons, and a ⅛-inch (3.18 mm) Rush awl and mallet. Have both racks of ³⁄₁₆-inch (4.76 mm) regular and looped condylar pins available (Fig. 5–22).
2. Place the anesthetized patient on the fracture table.
3. Adjust the knee rest under the fracture site and attach both feet in the foot plates firmly.

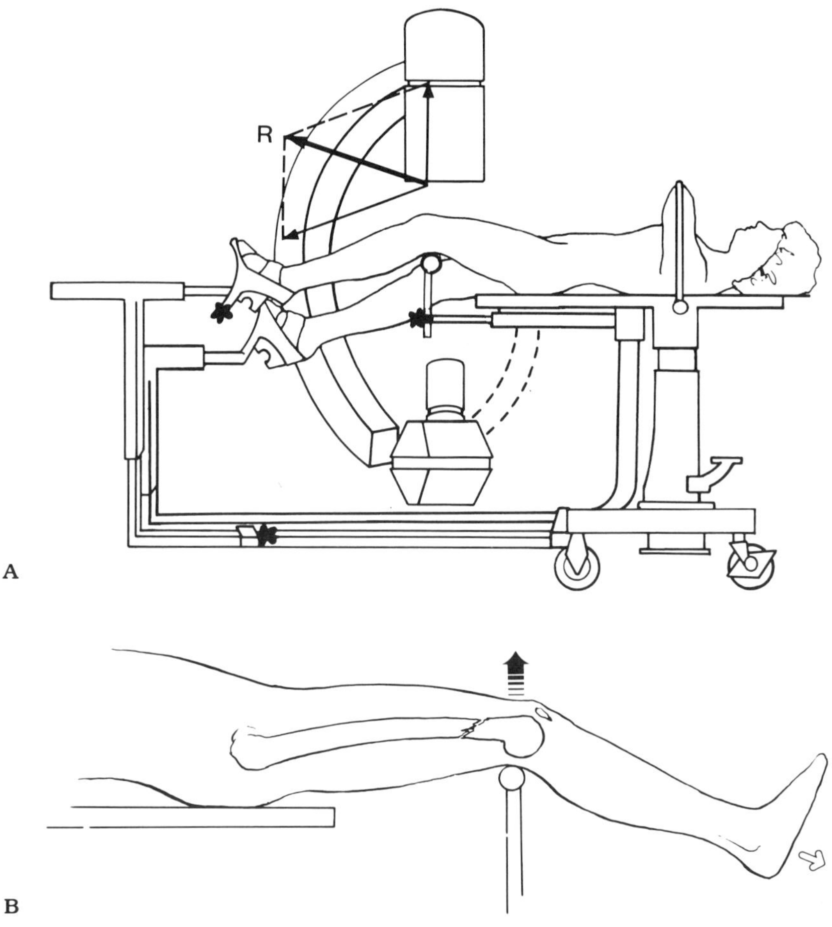

Figure 5–22.   (A) The limb on the fracture table is adjusted with the knee flexed and the countersupport at the fracture site. (B) Note change in the countersupport to reduce the supracondylar fracture.

4. Reduce the fracture by longitudinal traction, with the knee bent by manipulation over the knee rest that is positioned underneath the fracture so as to keep the femoral condyles from rotating posteriorly. Check the reduction with an image intensifier or regular anteroposterior and lateral radiographs (Fig. 5–22).

5–6. If the reduction is difficult, manual lateral pressure from the medial and lateral side should affect the overall alignment.

7. Prepare the skin surgically, preferably with alcohol and Ioban-II plastic drape that covers the distal part of the femur, the proximal part of the tibia, as well as the bar of the knee rest.

8. By using the image intensifier and awl as a pointer to find the level of the skin incision over the femoral condyles, make a skin incision 1 to 1½ inches (25–40 mm), through the skin capsule and into the joint all at once. The superior end of the incision should be approximately ¾ inch (2 cm) from the anterior and distal articular surfaces in line with the shaft of the femur (Fig. 5–23).

9. Put a ³⁄₁₆-inch (4.76 mm) Rush awl at the proximal end of the incision, at right angles to the condyles of the femur and perforate the cortex approximately ¼ inch (6 mm). This should give you an idea about the hardness of the condylar bone. For soft bone, you will need the looped condylar ³⁄₁₆-inch (4.76 mm) Rush pin. Medium hard bone can be handled with regular pins that are stress relieved, and for very hard bone in the young person, the straight regular ³⁄₁₆-inch (4.76 mm) Rush pins are adequate. With the cutting end of the awl in the direction of the shaft and a scooping motion, gradually cut away the distal bone until the awl is aimed at about 30 degrees to the long axis of the femur and exactly down the center in the lateral plane. The tip of the awl should be approximately 1 inch (2.5 cm) inside of the bone and directed to an imaginary point that the pin would cross the fracture site 3 to

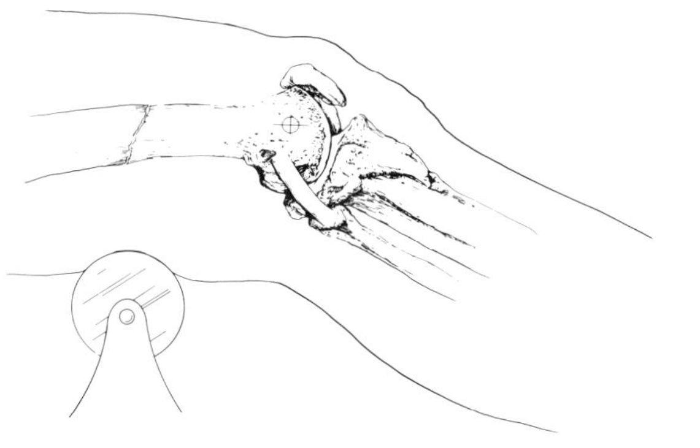

A

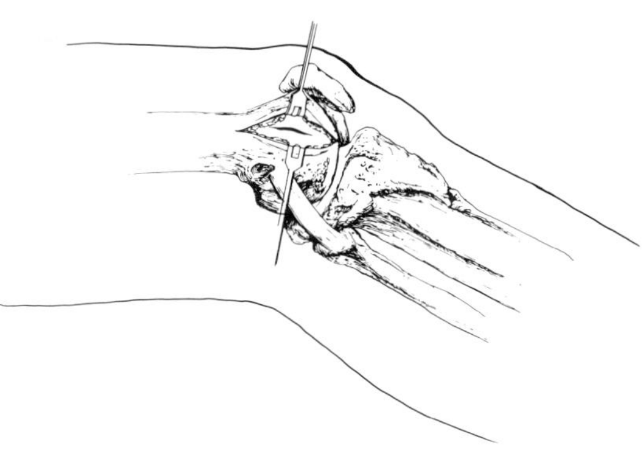

B

Figure 5–23. Location of skin incision in line with shaft of femur. **(A)** The fracture is reduced over the knee countersupport and the approach is made to the junction of the anterior one-third, posterior two-thirds of the femoral condyle, close to the articular surface. This point is in line with the midline of the femoral shaft. **(B)** The skin incision is made through skin subcutaneous tissue and joint capsule to expose the bone in this area.

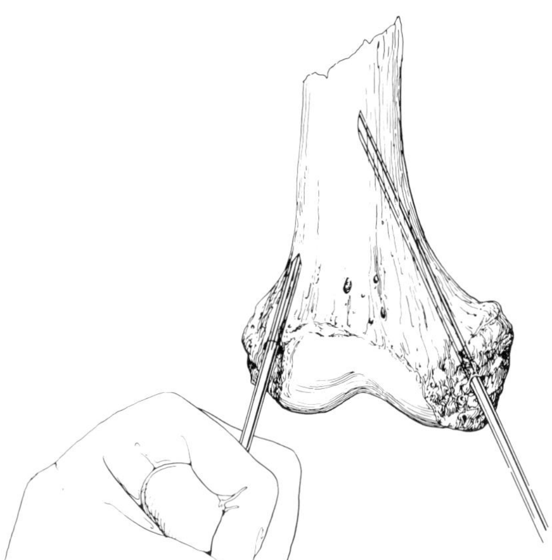

Figure 5–24.   The awl is inserted relatively close to the articular surface at right angles and then gradually moved with a cutting motion to aim toward the fracture surface, with the cutting slots still being able to cut the bone. A pin is inserted in one side while the other is prepared.

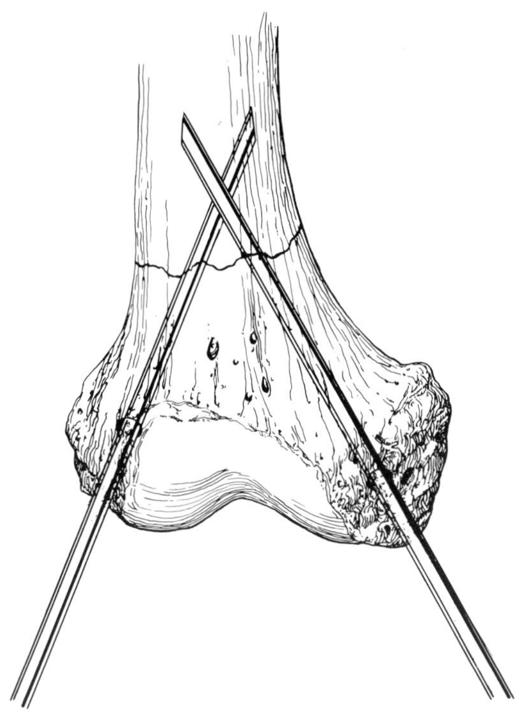

Figure 5–25.   The sled runner tips are turned so that the flat surfaces abut the inside cortex and slide up the medullary canal.

4 inches (8–10 cm) inside of the femur (Fig. 5–24).

10, 11. Put the sled runner tip of the straight ³⁄₁₆-inch (4.76 mm) C (24.13 cm) or D (26.04 cm) length Rush pin into the slot of the awl and introduce the pin into the femur approximately 2 inches (5 cm.) while removing the awl at the same time. Repeat the incision on the opposite condyle. Insert the awl in the same plane as the previously inserted pin that is projecting from the opposite side and then with a gradual scooping motion, change that direction so that it ends up in a 30-degree position to the long axis.

12. Do not bend pin.

13. Check the position by the image intensifier in anteroposterior and lateral directions.

14. Exchange the awl for another straight C or D length ³⁄₁₆-inch (4.76 mm) Rush pin.

15. Turn both sled runners about so that the flat surfaces of the sled runner may abut against the opposite cortex of the femur (Fig. 5–25).

16. Drive the pins up to the fracture site. If the fracture is transverse, either pin can be inserted across the fracture. Then the opposite pin can be placed across the fracture and the pins should be inserted deeply enough until they bounce off the opposite medullary cortex. At this time you will notice that the pins are more difficult to impact, as this is where the pin starts to get its gentle bend from the angle of insertion.

17. If the fracture is oblique, first insert the pin that is in the same line as the obliquity of the fracture, as it will always be the one that will be likely to exit the more proximal fracture site (Fig. 5–26).

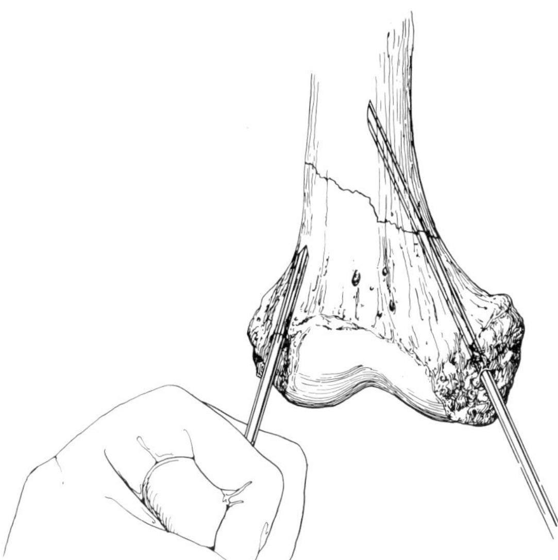

Figure 5–26. With an oblique fracture, the pin that would most likely go out of the fracture side is put across the fracture first, as the fracture is unstable and can be manipulated.

After the pin is up to the fracture site, manipulate the fracture by angulation or by use of the pin, and impact the sled runner across the fracture into the proximal fragment. At this time the second pin can be inserted across the fracture site with ease.

18. If the fracture has large comminuted pieces, that is, pieces longer than the diameter of the shaft, locate the center of these pieces by using the awl as a pointer and the image intensifier and then make an anterolateral incision through the fascia to expose the femur slightly. Pass No. 16 or 18 malleable stainless-steel wires around the femur with a wire passer, without stripping the muscle away from the fragments. Tighten the wire to tubulate the bone. Usually one or two cerclage wires is sufficient. After tubulation of the femur, first insert the pin which is most likely to come out of the comminuted fractures into

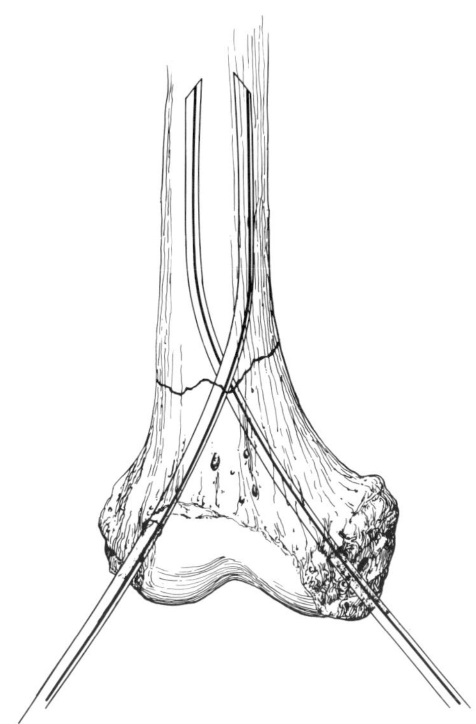

Figure 5–27. After the straight ³⁄₁₆-inch (4.76 cm) Rush pins have crossed the supracondylar fracture and the sled runners abut the inside of the medullary canal, the pins will be advanced alternately and will start to develop a curve. As the pins develop a curve, there is an increase in stability at the fracture site and the sound of impaction.

the proximal fragment, and then alternately impact the pins until the sled runners are inside the proximal medullary canal.

19. After the sled runners are in the proximal part of the medullary canal, alternately impact the pins until 3 to 4 inches (8 to 10 cm) are left outside of the bone. This is the time to stress relieve the pins if the bone is soft or moderately soft (Fig. 5–27). By radiographic viewing, at this time, the straight pins will have started to bend inside of the femur and the surgeon will notice that the impaction of the pins has become more difficult.

20. Stress relieve the ³⁄₁₆-inch (4.76 cm) Rush pin by using a bending

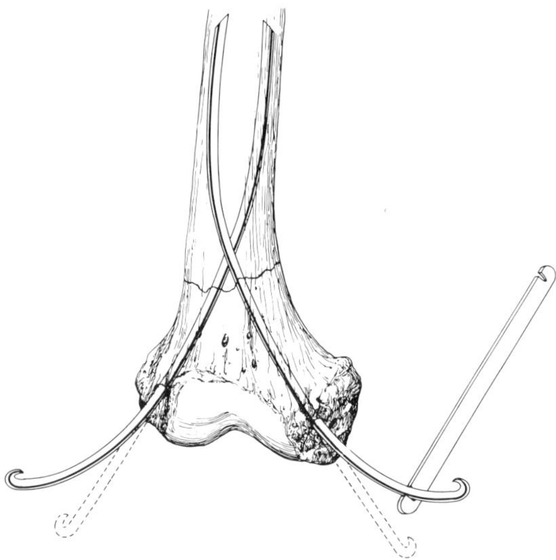

Figure 5–28. In soft condylar bone, the pins are stress relieved to prevent inward migration, by putting in more permanent bend in the last few inches with the bending irons.

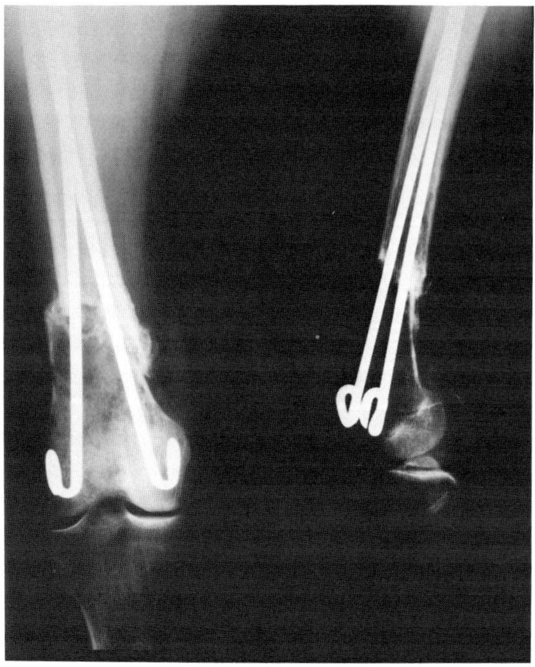

Figure 5–29. Looped condylar pins in pathologic fracture. A 72-year-old woman had a pathologic fracture of the distal end of the femur above the condyles. The patient had diagnosed adenocarcinoma in the spine and ribs. After the fracture was reduced on the fracture table with the countersupport and awl holes were made in the proper direction, one awl was removed and a long pituitary rongeur was placed in the medullary canal and a biopsy specimen obtained. The hole was then filled with a looped condylar pin, which was inserted in the usual manner and contoured to fit the femoral condyles. Radiation therapy to the femur and spine was started within the week.

iron in one hand and the femur in the other (Fig. 5–28). Move the site of the bending iron on the Rush pin to different spots so that the bend in the pin is gradual. Stress relieving must not be so much that the pin, when inserted, does not cause pressure against the more centrally located bone.

21. Use the impactor to insert the pin head underneath the capsule of the joint so that the head of the pin is just visible and tends to grip the femoral cortex. If the loop condylar pins are used, when the pinhead is about 1 inch from the medial or lateral femoral cortex, observe the plane of the femoral condyle and you will notice that the lateral femoral condyle is almost vertical and the medial one is much more oblique. Use the narrow end of the Rush bending iron to fit over the flattened looped condylar head of the pin and bend the loop so that it will eventually lay parallel to the condylar surface. Then impact the head, inserting the looped head underneath the capsule (Fig. 5–29). In hard bone, without stress relieving, the pins will have a gentle curve when viewed with the image intensifier at this stage.

22. Release the traction, if using the fracture table, and observe the fracture and the head of the pin. They should not back out. If they tend to do this, back the pins out and change the degree of stress relieving of the pin with the bending iron.

23. Use heavy suture to close the

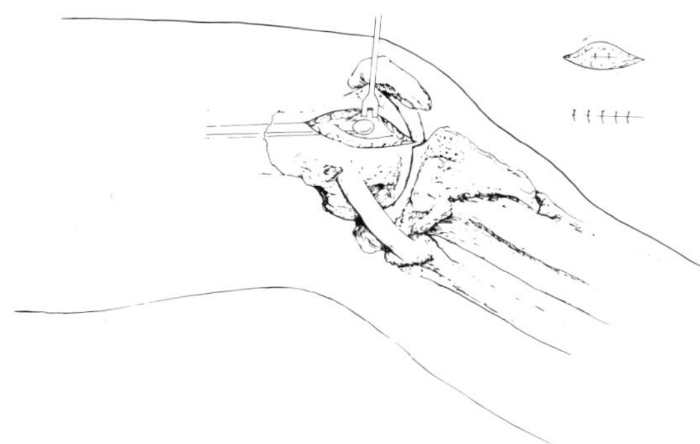

Figure 5–30. After the pin is seated in the bone, the capsule is closed over the head of the pin so that the pin can slide under the capsule and give knee support.

capsule over the pin head and put the knee through a range of motion. If motion stops at 30 degrees of flexion, the head of the pin must be protruding through the fascia of the capsule, and this must be corrected (Fig. 5–30).

24. A postoperative knee splint can be used until the patient has returned to the room, and active knee motion can be started as soon as the wound permits (Figs. 5–31, 5–32).

Femoral Condyles: T or Y Supracondylar Fracture

Fixation of a T or Y fracture of a femoral condyle (Fig. 5–33) becomes more complex, but is dealt with by using the same basic principles as described already. On the fracture table with the knee support, the fracture is reduced as best as possible with the traction and manipulation. Incisions are made on both sides of the femoral condyles as before, and an awl, ³⁄₁₆ inch (4.76 cm) in size, is used to penetrate each of the condyles. This allows the awl to be used as a manipulator and align the joint surface. After the T or Y fragment has been aligned, a ⅛-inch (3.18 cm) long awl can be placed through the condyles from lateral to medial to stabilize

the fractures. Then the ³⁄₁₆-inch (4.76 cm) Rush pins can be inserted across the fractures into the medullary canal. Refer to Flow Sheet on page 29.

The Y fractures (Fig. 5–34) can be manipulated using the awls that have not gone to the fracture line, to reduce the interarticular condyles as seen with the image intensifier.

After the reduction of the fracture, an awl can be placed across the condyles. This will temporarily hold the condyles in position. The awl can be exchanged with a ⅛-inch (3.18 mm) pin if necessary; however, the resilient forces of the pins frequently squeeze the condyles together so tightly that the pin becomes long and has to be exchanged (Fig. 5–35).

As the straight pins develop a curve, the compressive force between the T or Y fragments increases and stability improves (Figs. 5–35, 5–36).

Subtrochanteric Fracture

The subtrochanteric region should be approached cautiously. (Refer to the Flow Sheet on page 29.) In young people, the greater trochanter is firm cancellous bone and can hold the fixation well. In older people, the bone is less firm and fixation can be tenuous.

Two absolute contraindications to pinning are a stiff hip usually due to arthritis and fracture lines extending from the subtrochanteric area into the trochanters. If these are present, some other method of treatment is advisable, usually a prosthetic replacement.

This type of fracture frequently results in nonunion because of the muscle pull forces and the narrow cortical canal. Cancellous bone grafting, therefore, is advisable at the time of surgery.

The ¼-inch (6.35 mm) awl can be used for direction of the Ender pin since one pin is all that will usually fit into the medullary canal of young people.

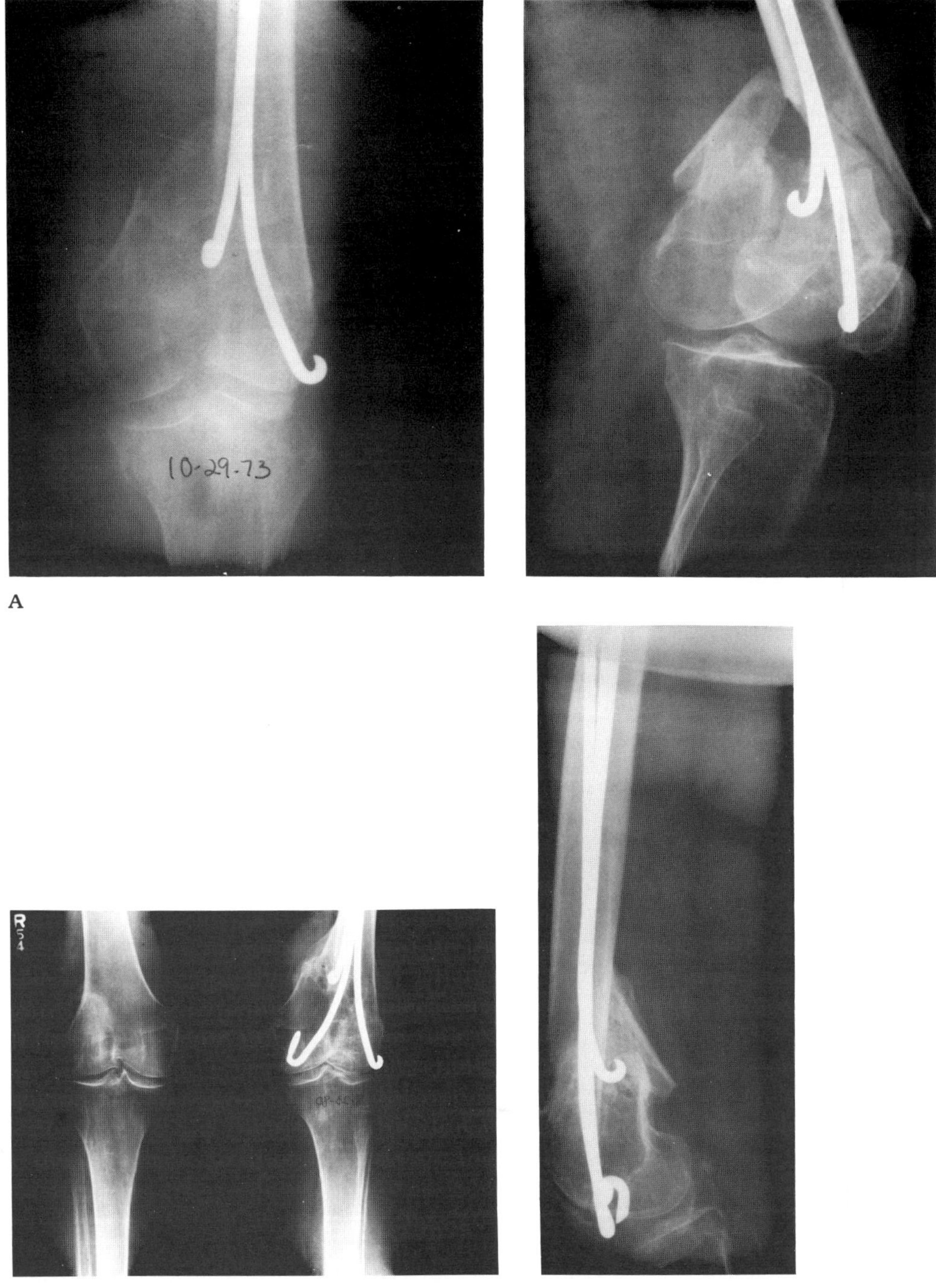

Figure 5–31. Effects of stress-relieving and looped condylar pins in soft bone. **(A)** A 72-year-old female pharmacist fell at her store. At the first surgery, the soft bone was not appreciated and the medial pin was only slightly stress relieved. Within 3 days, the pin migrated into the medullary canal as seen and fixation was tenuous. **(B)** The patient was returned to surgery and a looped condylar pin was inserted in the same general area, with no attempt to get the disappeared pin. The looped condylar pin was also stress relieved. The fracture promptly healed, and the patient returned to her work in 3 months. Follow-up 7 years later with standing radiographs revealed no arthritic change and a well-healed fracture with three intramedullary Rush pins.

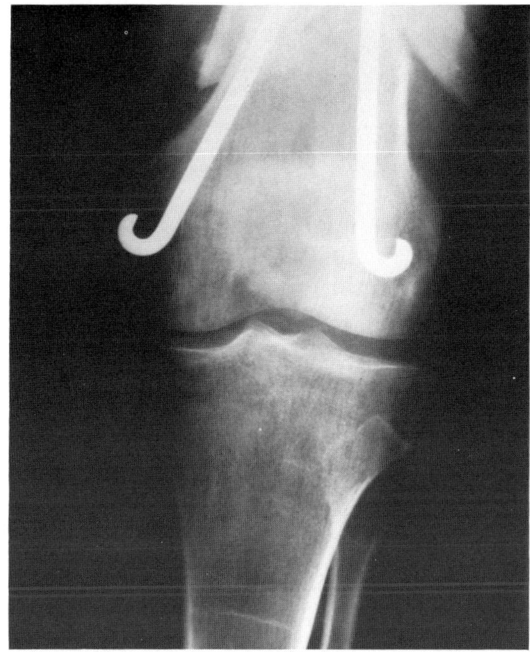

A

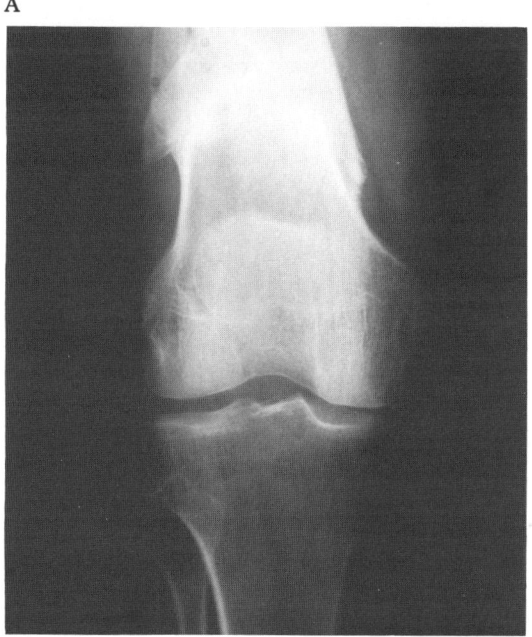

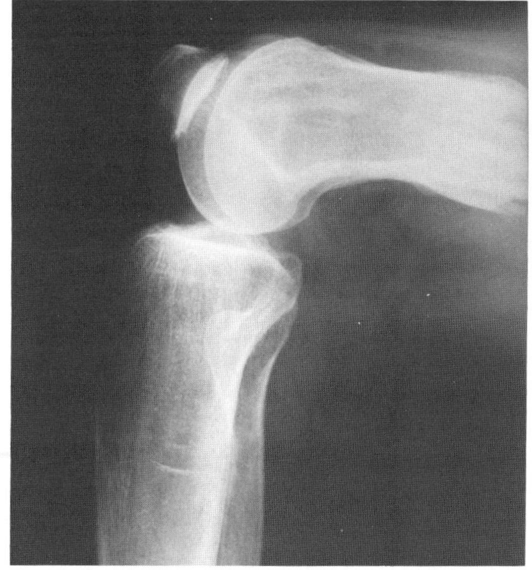

B

Figure 5–32. Comminuted fracture not treated with cerclage wire. (**A**) A 59-year-old man with comminuted supracondylar fracture of the femur. Two pins were inserted without cerclage wires, and the cancellous bone promptly healed. (**B**) Radiographs were taken at 7 months, and the pins were removed.

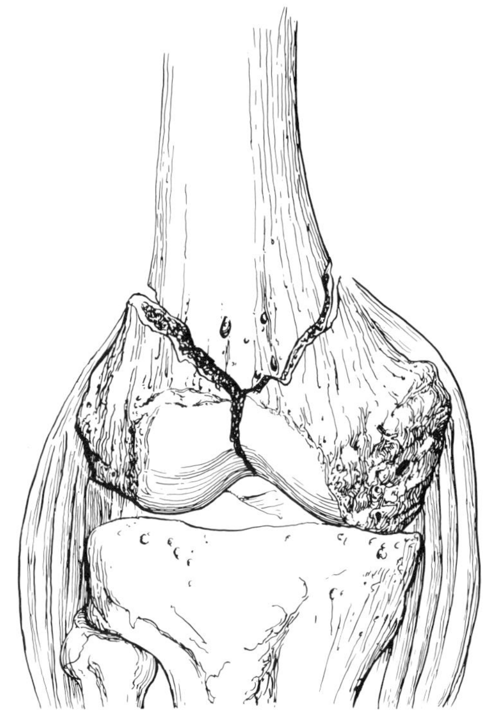

Figure 5–33.   Y-type supracondylar fracture.

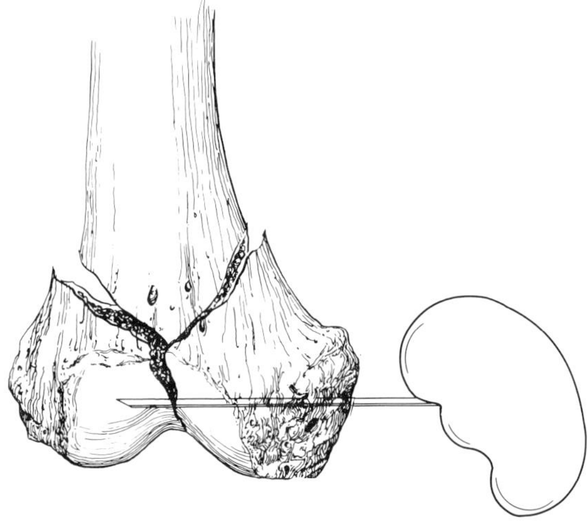

Figure 5–34.   The awl into each condylar fracture can reduce the fracture, and then a smaller awl can be placed across the condyles to hold them until the ³⁄₁₆-inch (4.76 mm) resilient pins can compress and hold the fractures.

1. Have the necessary rack of special ¼-inch (6.35 mm) shepherd's crook Rush pins, cerclage wire, wire tighteners, wire passers, and Ender pins, as well as the other Rush and Ender instruments.
2. Place the anesthetized patient on the fracture table.
3. Place traction on both legs, with the uninjured leg in slight extension at the hip. Fasten both feet to the foot plates.
4. Place the knee rest under the affected thigh, with the leg slightly adducted and the hip slightly flexed.
5. Observe the position of the fracture with the image intensifier and manipulate the fracture. If the reduction is easy, the awl can be introduced into the greater trochanter tip more medially and at about a 10 to 20-degree angle to the shaft (Fig. 5–37).
6. If the reduction is difficult, the awl may have to be placed in the fracture site and aimed to exit laterally in the area of the greater trochanter.
7. Prepare and drape the skin. Be sure to cover the buttocks and proximal area of the hip with Ioban-II drape.
8. Make two incisions: one in the midlateral area over the greater trochanter going more proximally down to the fracture site, and the second at the level of the adductor tubercle, slightly anterior to it.
9. A ¼-inch (6.35 mm) Rush awl is started at the top of the greater trochanter in the gluteus medius, aiming at a 10 to 20-degree angle toward the fracture site.
10. The adductor tubercle region is approached with an Ender awl and a hole of an appropriate size is made gently, changing the align-

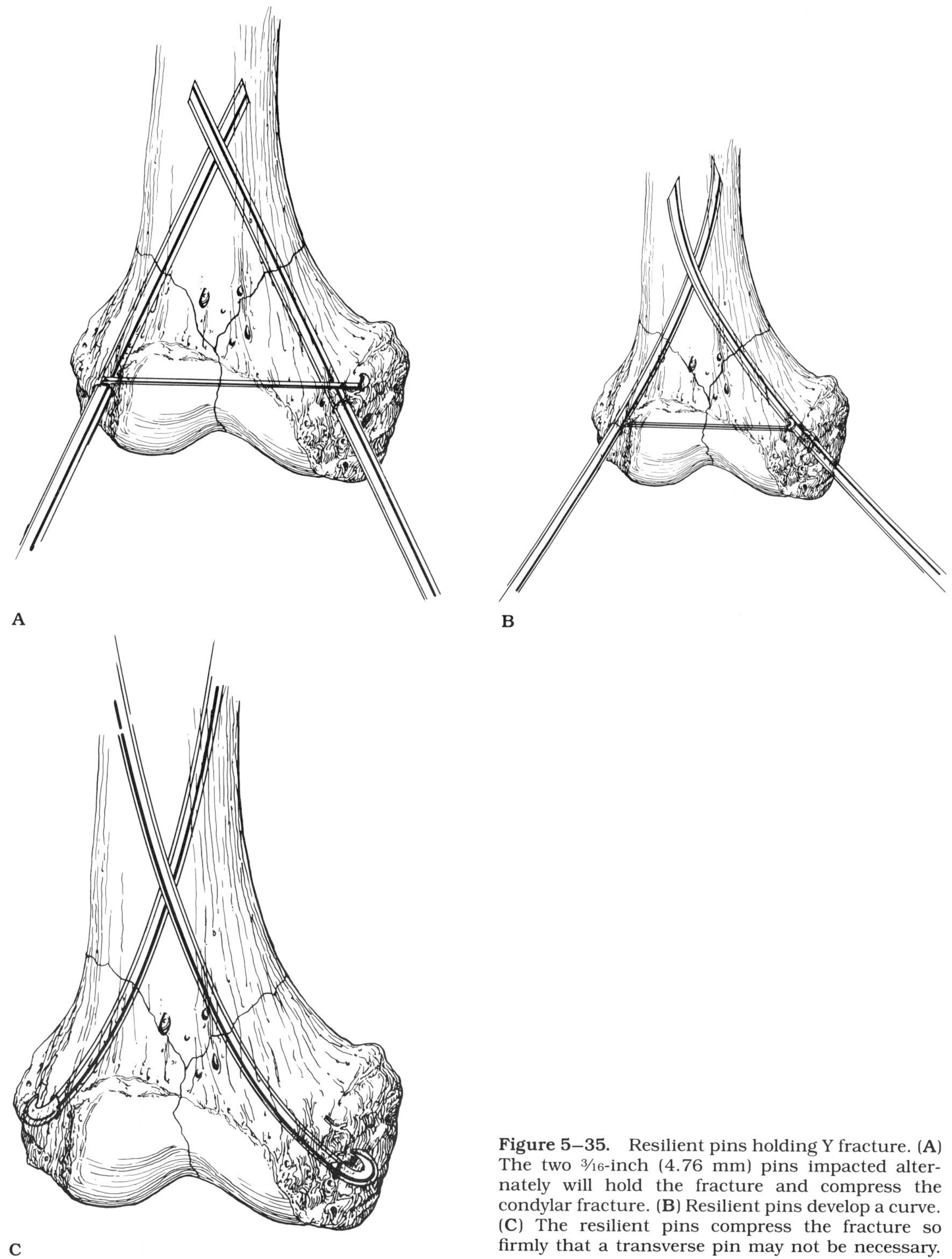

Figure 5–35.   Resilient pins holding Y fracture. (**A**) The two ³⁄₁₆-inch (4.76 mm) pins impacted alternately will hold the fracture and compress the condylar fracture. (**B**) Resilient pins develop a curve. (**C**) The resilient pins compress the fracture so firmly that a transverse pin may not be necessary.

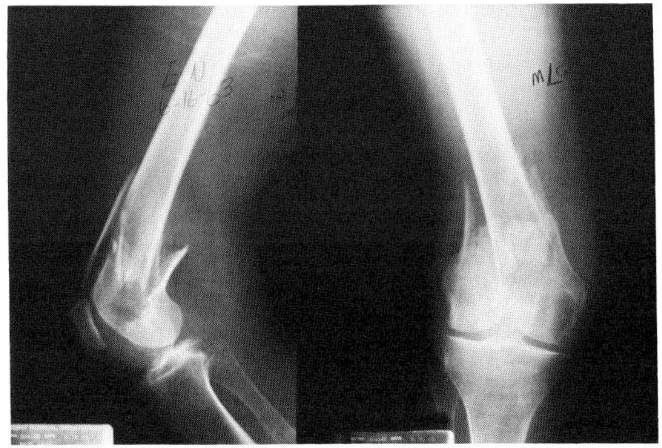

A

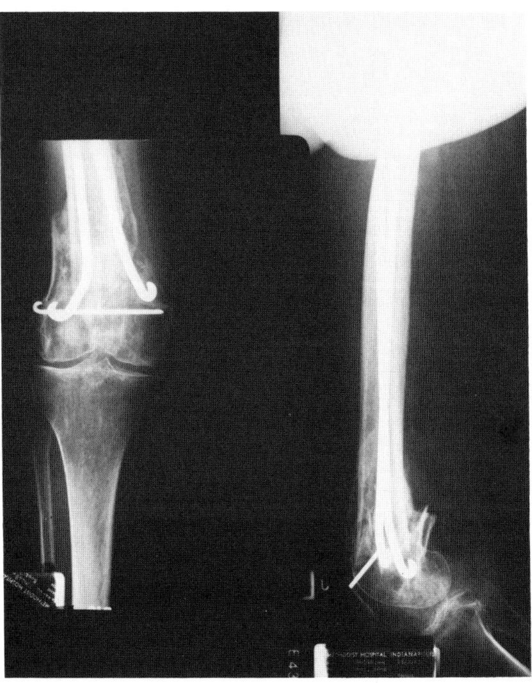

B

Figure 5–36. Healing in a short supracondylar fracture. **(A)** A 76-year-old woman who had a short comminuted supracondylar fracture pinned in a closed fashion. **(B)** The fracture healed within 5 months with full weight-bearing.

ment so that the awl points up the shaft of the femur.

11. Determine the length of the shepherd's crook pins to be used by measuring from the top of the trochanter to the adductor tubercle region.

12. Bend the shepherd's crook pin into a gentle curve that is appropriate for the size of the medullary canal. Generally, older people have a wider medullary canal and need a greater bend.

13. If it is a comminuted or a spiral fracture, cerclage wires are used at this time, with minimal stripping of the soft tissues at the fracture site.

14. Exchange the pin for the awl and with visualization by the image intensifier, pound the pin down to the fracture site.

15. Use the pin to manipulate the proximal part of the femur and help guide the pin into the distal end. If cerclage wires are used, they must be tightened appropriately at this time, to tubulate the bone.

16–20. Go to the knee incision and measure the appropriate length for an Ender pin that will go into the middle area of the neck. Insert the Ender pin up to the fracture site in the usual method. Manipulate both of the pins so that they can go into the opposite medullary canal without inserting them too deeply (Fig. 5–37). Impact the shepherd's crook pin so it engages the bone substance of the greater trochanter and its distal top is in the lateral femoral condyle.

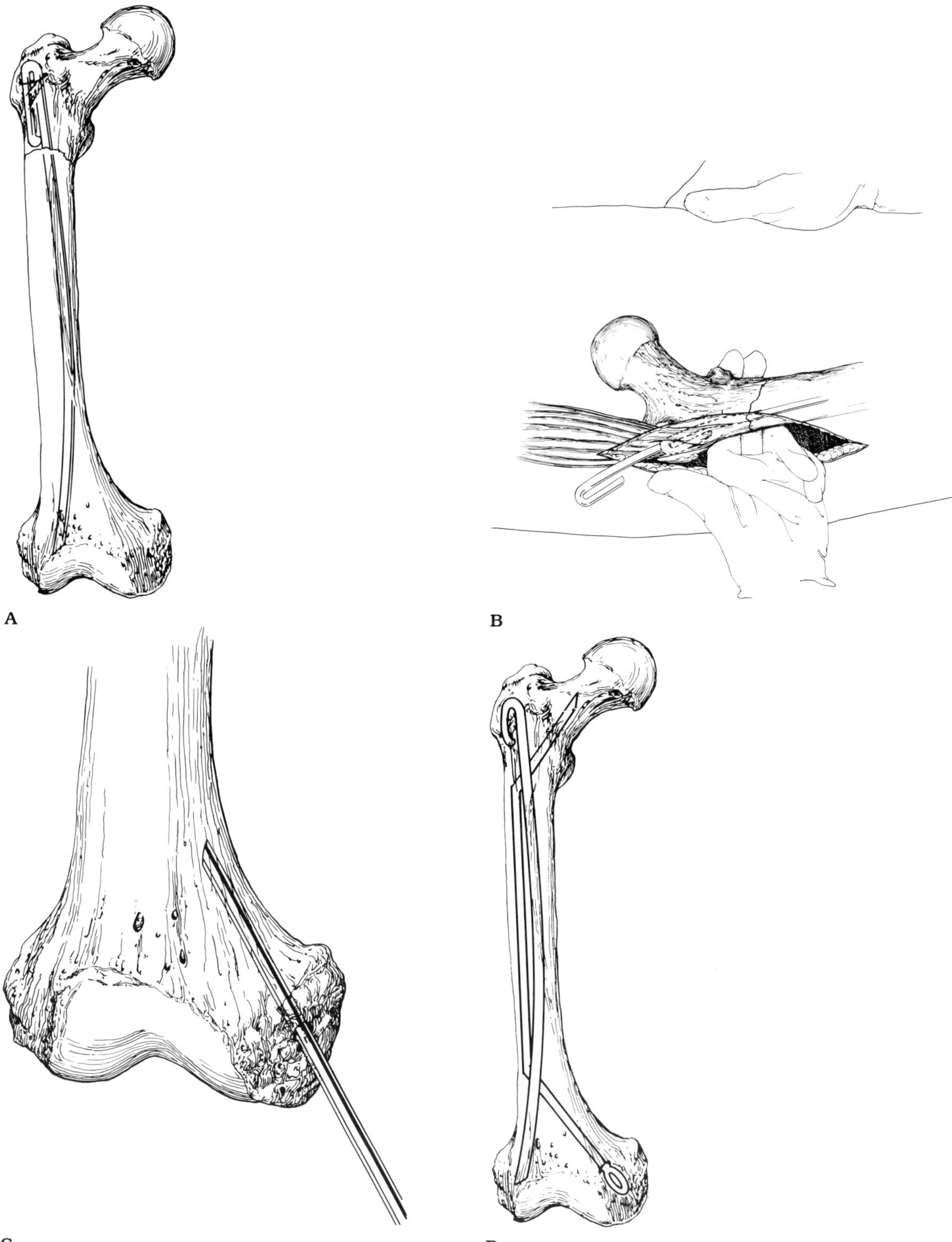

Figure 5–37. Subtrochanteric fracture. (**A**) A shepherd's crook ¼inch (6.35 mm) pin is prebent and inserted more medially in the trochanter. (Usually this is not a satisfactory enough fixation.) (**B**) The shepherd's crook pin is placed across the fracture and seated by the semi-open or open technique. The hook is impacted into the greater trochanter. (**C**) A ¼-inch (6.35 mm) awl hole is made into the medial femoral condyle for insertion of an Ender pin. (**D**) The combination of the shepherd's crook and the Ender pin gives good fixation with a minimum of trauma in surgery.

21. Insert the Ender pin so that the tip of the pin is in the midportion of the neck of the femur.

22, 23. Loosen the traction, impact both of the pins, and observe it under the image intensifier.

24. Routine closure of the wounds and placement of a suction drain in the area of the fracture is important.

25, 26. Remove the patient from the fracture table and place in bed, with the hip and knee in a flexed position (Fig. 5–38).

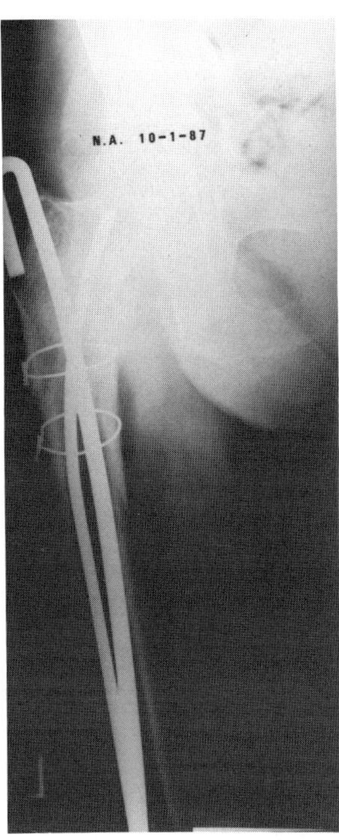

Figure 5–38. An 80-year-old demented woman fell at the nursing home and suffered a spiral closed subtrochanteric hip fracture. The fracture was reduced on the Rush table. Two cerclage wires were passed and tightened while a precurved shepherd's crook Rush pin was inserted from the greater trochanter and seated. An Ender pin inserted through a ³⁄₁₆-inch (4.76 mm) awl hole on the medial femoral condyle was placed across the spiral fracture into the neck without difficulty, using image intensification control. Walker training was attempted, but was not successful as the patient could not remember how to use the walker. The fracture was healed at 4 months in spite of her efforts to climb out of bed and walk on it.

Fractures at the Junction of Distal and Middle Thirds

Displacement of fractures at the junction of the distal and middle thirds is similar, but less marked than in the supracondylar area. Reduction is accomplished as with fractures in the shaft or supracondylar area by using the countersupport on the table. Fixation is difficult because of the shape of the bone and healing is the slowest, usually associated with inadequate fixation using a single pin or lack of cerclage wires, or both (Fig. 5–40).

1. Have the necessary ¼-inch (6.35 mm) and ³⁄₁₆-inch (4.76 mm) Rush pins and appropriate Rush instruments.

2. Place the anesthetized patient on the fracture table and fasten both feet to the foot plates.

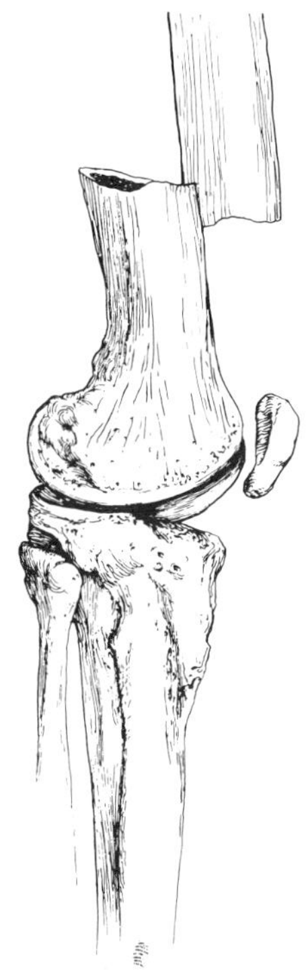

Figure 5–39. Fractures of the trumpet-shaped distal third of the femoral shaft are difficult to hold with intramedullary fixation.

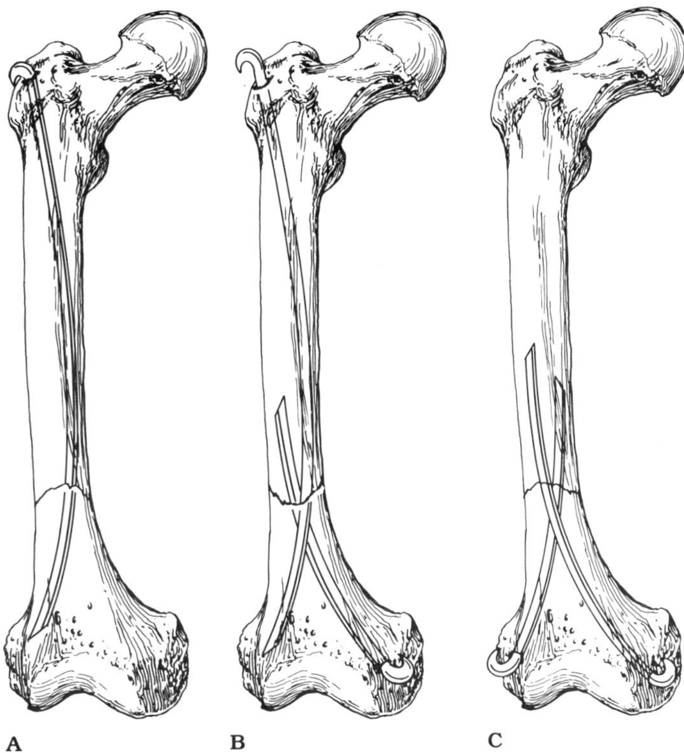

Figure 5–40. Three methods of fixation of the distal third of the femoral shaft. (**A**) Fixation with a single pin from the greater trochanter usually does not provide sufficient support for the fracture, as does single insertion from the lateral condyle. (**B**) Two-pin fixation gives the best fixation combining static a precurved ¼-inch (6.35 mm) pin used for shaft fractures with a dynamically curved ³⁄₁₆-inch (4.76 mm) pin driven from the medial femoral condyle. (**C**) Occasionally straight ³⁄₁₆-inch (4.76 mm) pins can be placed across the fracture in a closed fashion and give excellent fixation.

A　　　　B　　　　C

3. Put traction on both legs, with the unaffected limb and hip in slight extension.
4. Adjust the knee rest at this time.
5. Manipulate the femur by adjusting the height of the knee rest and the amount of traction and by side to side manipulation. Check it with the image intensifier.
6. Difficult reductions may need the use of a crutch and strap but one should try to have the fracture reducible at this time.
7. Prepare the skin in the usual manner, from the hip to below the knee circumferentially, and use sterile drapes.
8. Two incisions are needed: The trochanteric approach is the same as with the closed femoral shaft fractures, and the medial approach is the same as with supracondylar fractures.
9. Start the ¼-inch (6.35 mm) awl at

right angles to the shaft at the level of the greater trochanter to find out how hard the bone is to penetrate. Then by a gentle scooping action, adjust the ¼-inch (6.35 mm) awl to a 30-degree angle to the long axis of the shaft of the femur.

10. With the ³⁄₁₆-inch (4.76 mm) awl make an initial hole at right angles to the medial femoral condyle and gradually angle the awl to 30-degree angle to the long axis of the femur in the anteroposterior plane and in exactly the same line in the lateral plane.
11. Measure the length of the ¼-inch (6.35 mm) pin. This length is critical, for the ¼-inch (6.35 mm) pin should go deep into the femoral condyle and should end up usually at the same level as the insertion of the ³⁄₁₆ (5–10 cm) awl hole. A ³⁄₁₆-inch (4.76 mm) pin

should go 2 to 4 inches (5–10 cm) into the proximal part of the medullary canal.

12. With a bending iron prebend the ¼-inch (6.35 mm) pin into a gentle bend. Young people with small medullary canals take less of a gentle bend than elderly people with wide medullary canals. Use the image to see whether the curve is sufficient. The curve will usually shorten the pin about one pin size length, and the tip should be at the level of the midcondyle when bent. The ³⁄₁₆-inch (4.76 mm) pin should not be prebent on a general basis.

13. Check the angles of the awl with relationship to the long axis of the femur.

14. Exchange the awl for a ¼-inch (6.35 mm) Rush pin by sliding the sled runner tip in the awl slot so that it engages the bone. Do the same with the ³⁄₁₆-inch (4.76 mm) pin from the medial side of the knee.

15. Turn both of the sled runners around so that the sled runner faces the opposite medullary cortex.

16. Impact a ¼-inch (6.35 mm) pin just to the fracture line.

17. Under the image intensifier, manipulate the pin and the femur so that the pin can be inserted across the fracture site.

18. Place the distal fragment in varus stress by manipulation at the fracture site and at the knee. Then

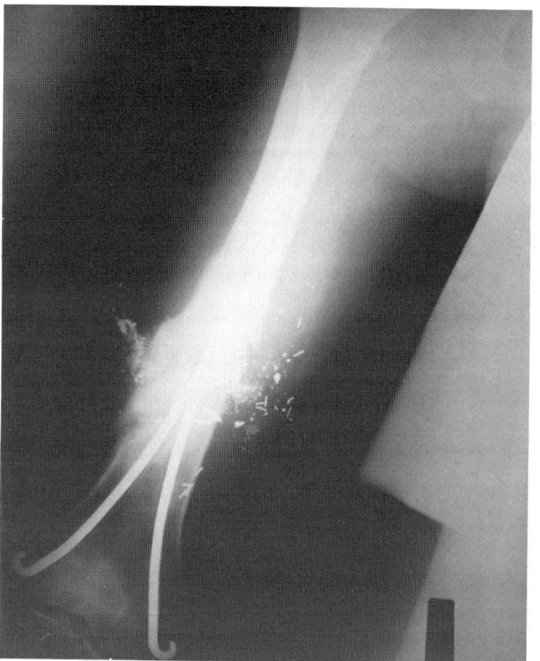
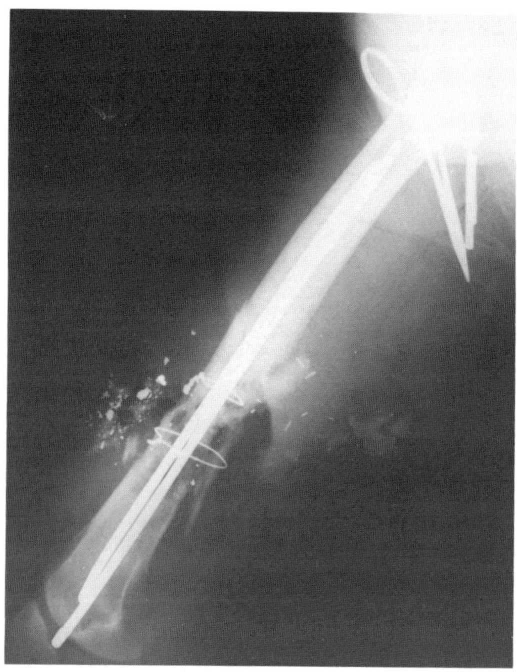

Figure 5–41.   Open fractures of the femur. A 24-year-old man had a gunshot wound and Gustilo Grade III fracture at the junction of the middle and distal third. Immediate debridement, arterial repair, and cerclage wiring preceded the arterial repair on November 19, 1986. A follow-up radiograph showed a healed fracture on May 19, 1987. Two ³⁄₁₆ inch (4.76 mm) Rush pins were used. The pins were bent near their tip for getting across the fracture site. Fortunately, the medullary canal was wide enough so that the pins did not catch in the medullary canal and prevent seating the pins.

impact the pin so that the tip ends up in the lateral femoral condyle.

19,20. Insert the ³⁄₁₆-inch (4.76 mm) straight Rush pin across the fracture site and 3 to 4 inches (7–10 cm) into the proximal part. Infrequently, it will be necessary to prebend the ³⁄₁₆-inch (4.76 mm) pin.

21–23. Check both views with an image intensifier and be very careful that there is no distraction at the fracture site. It is generally a good idea to loosen the traction at this time.

24. Close the incisions, being careful at the knee to have the capsule sutured over the pins that have been seated.

25,26. If this is the only fracture, hold the knee in an anterior plaster splint, with the knee at right angle so that the knee can be elevated until the swelling goes down (Figs. 5–41, 5–42, 5–43).

Condyle Fractures

Fracture of the femoral condyle requires accurate reduction because it goes through the articular surface. This is usually best done with the leg over the countersupport and in traction. An incision on the side of the fracture, using a ³⁄₁₆-inch (4.76 mm) awl to help in the reduction, will usually be sufficient. After reduction, maintenance of the reduction can be done with a ⅛-inch (3.18 mm) awl going to the opposite condyle and then the ³⁄₁₆-inch (4.76 mm) pin can be dynamically impacted to hold the femur stable.

Occasionally with severely comminuted supracondylar fractures, a portion of the medial or lateral femoral condyle is fractured away. This is usually below insertion of the gastrocnemius and a single straight ⅛-inch (3.18 mm) pin, used as a dynamic pin inserted at the edge of the articular surface and bouncing off the opposite cortex, will provide sufficient stability of the fracture so that active motion at the knee can be started at an early time (Figs. 5–44, 5–45, 5–46, 5–47).

The Rush fracture table with the bilateral offset countersupports or knee rests is particularly helpful in the treatment of bilateral fractures of the femoral shaft in the multiple trauma or polytrauma patient. Countersupports are at different levels so that the lateral radiograph of the more distal fracture is easy to discern. The countersupport is a rounded horizontal bar, attached to the table under the perineal post, which is placed under the limb at varying locations to reduce the fracture. It is used in conjunction with fraction forces. The most distal of the fractures distal fracture should be on the countersupport that is the most elevated. This makes lateral radiographs easy to obtain (Fig. 5–48).

PITFALLS

All of the basic techniques discussed in Chapter 4 are applicable to fractures of the femur using a static ¼-inch (6.35 mm) pin inserted from either the lateral femoral condyle or the greater trochanter. Three-sixteenth-inch (4.76 mm) resilient straight pins can be inserted from the supracondylar area or a combination of both a ³⁄₁₆- (4.76 mm) and a ¼inch (6.35 mm) pin with the use of bending irons to preshape the pins can be used as mentioned in this chapter. One of the pitfalls that is seen in the patient who has a fracture treated with Rush pins is when there is no rapid formation of callus. The most frequent site of this problem is the junction of the middle and distal thirds of the femur. If callus does not occur rapidly, the development of a nonunion should be deemed to be almost imminent unless the

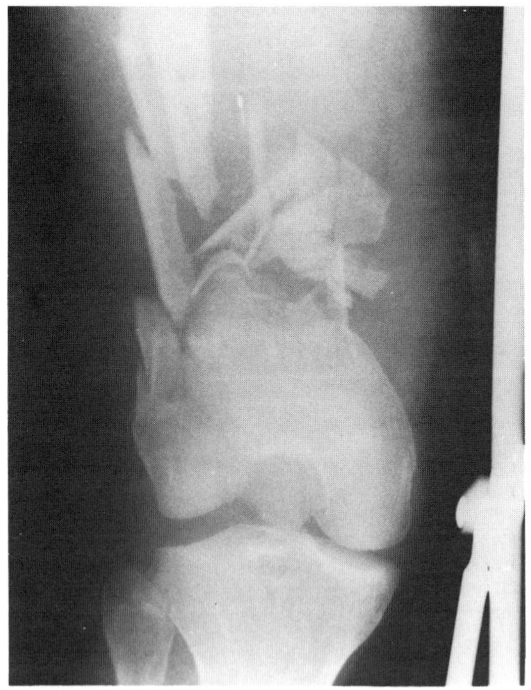

A

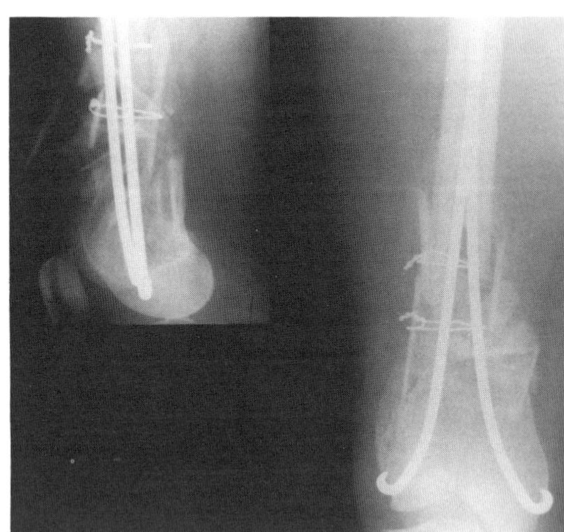

B

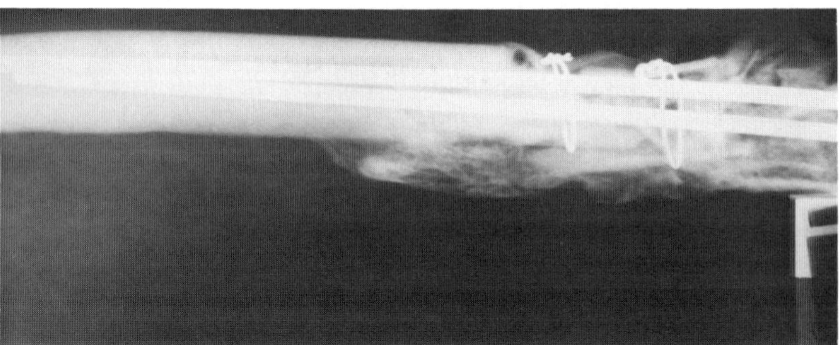

C

Figure 5–42.   Comminuted supracondylar fracture and fracture of the distal third (**A**) A 54-year-old woman involved in an automobile accident had a comminuted displaced fracture in the distal part of the femur treated in skeletal traction for a week. The fracture was reduced on a Rush table, but the comminuted split fractures could not be retubulated completely because of the abundant callus, even in this short time. (**B**) Two ³⁄₁₆-inch (4.76 mm) straight pins were passed into the proximal part of the shaft and fixation with cerclage wires was attempted; however, they could not be passed around all of the fracture, and the lateral wires were passed around the fracture and the medial intramedullary Rush pin. A knee immobilizer was applied for 6 weeks. (**C**) Fracture healing at 4½ months showed abundant callus formation, including endosteal callus, even where periosteum is not noted (continued).

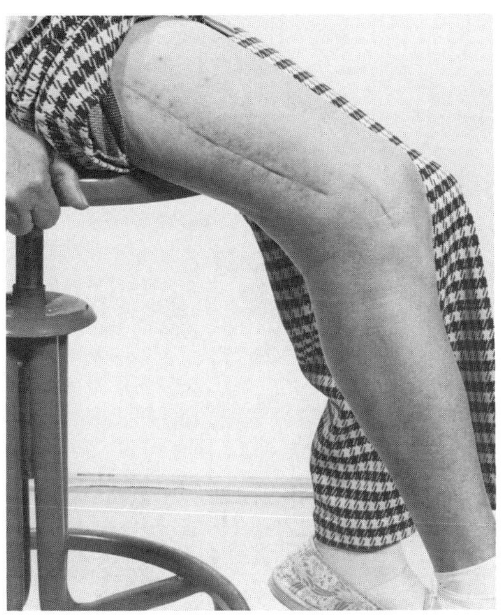

D

Figure 5–42 (cont.).   (D) Maximum flexion of 52 degrees is noted at the 1 year follow-up. The majority of the loss of motion can be attributed to comminuted fracture; however, a straight lateral approach makes the cerclage wiring much more difficult and probably helps with adherence of the soft tissues to the fascia lata.

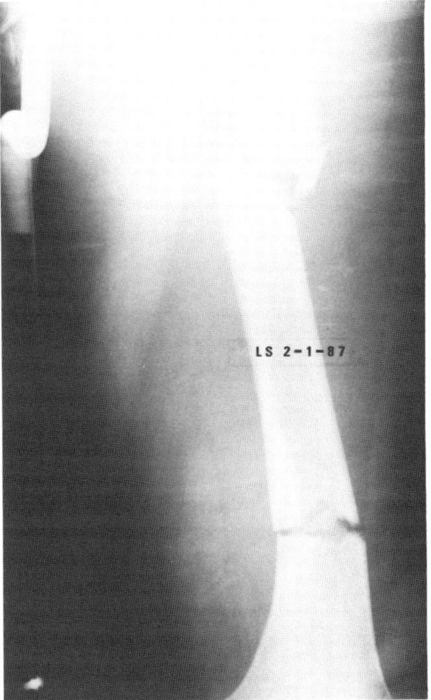

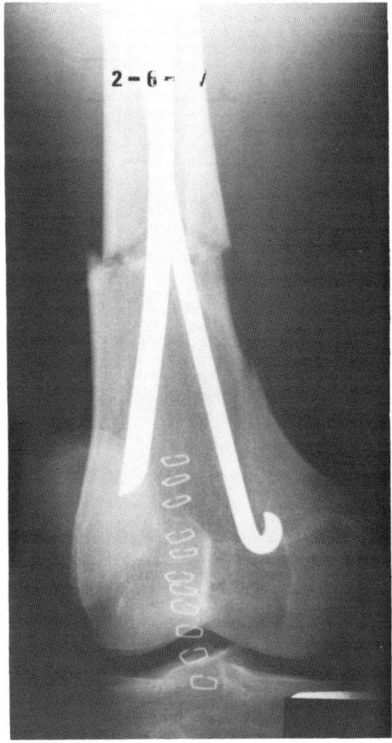

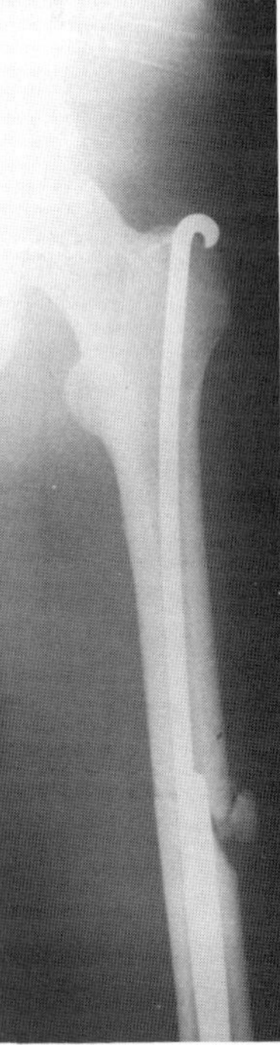

A

B

Figure 5–43.   (A) A 21-year-old man had a closed segmental femoral fracture at the isthmus of the femur and approximately 5 inches (12.5 cm) above the femoral articular surface. (B) The fracture was reduced on the fracture table with traction and the use of the countersupport and knee rest. The proximal ¼-inch (6.35 mm) pin was slightly curved due to the narrow femoral canal, and by twisting the head appropriately, the pin transversed both fractures in a closed fashion and ended in the lateral femoral condyle. A straight ³⁄₁₆-inch (4.76 mm) pin was inserted from the medial femoral condyle to provide additional stability because of the flared medullary canal.

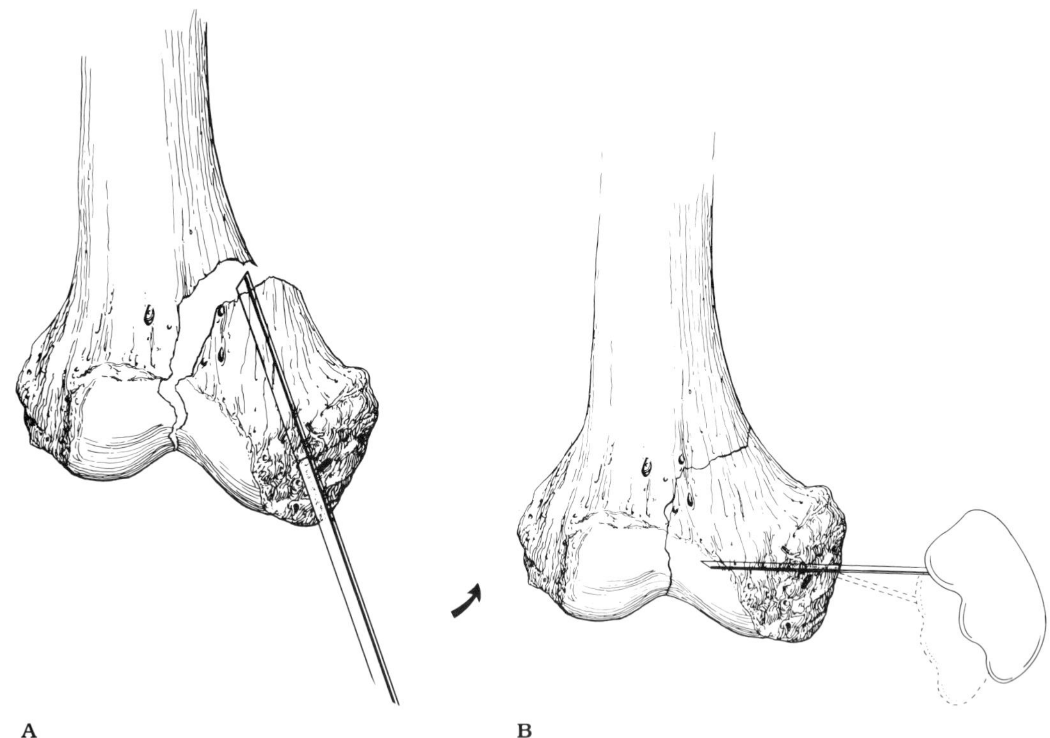

Figure 5–44.   A single condyle fracture. (**A**) Single condylar fractures are frequently displaced by a muscle pull, usually the gastrocnemius. Reduction is somewhat possible on the fracture table, but displacement is always present. (**B**) A ³⁄₁₆-inch (4.76 mm) awl can spear the fragment through a single incision and the awl can be used to direct the fracture and close up the fracture line.

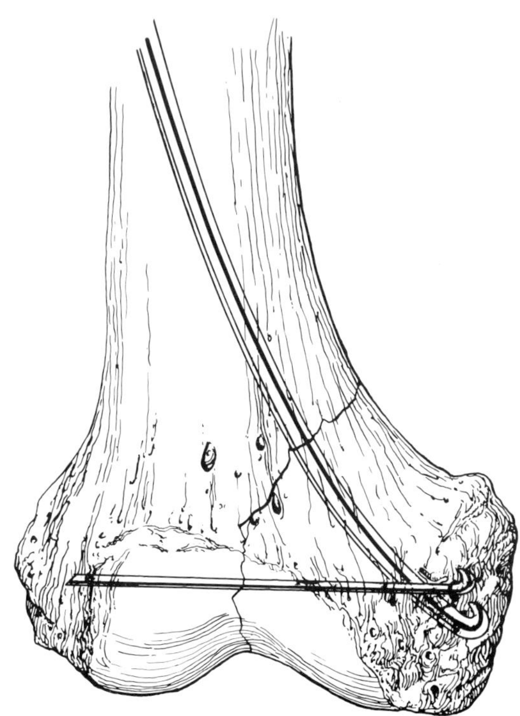

Figure 5–45.   After the reduction with the awl, a ⅛-inch (3.18 mm) awl can be placed across the fracture line and a ³⁄₁₆-inch (4.76 mm) pin and ⅛-inch (3.18 mm) pin to pin this fracture. A ³⁄₁₆-inch (4.76 mm) pin inserted straight produces the vector force to close the fracture and the alignment is maintained with a short ⅛-inch pin. Early motion can be started in this situation.

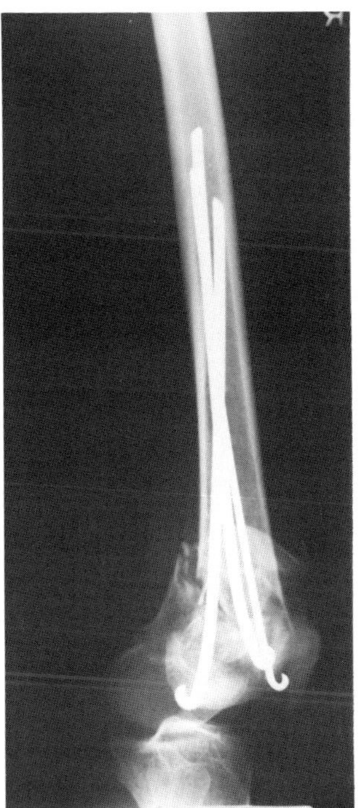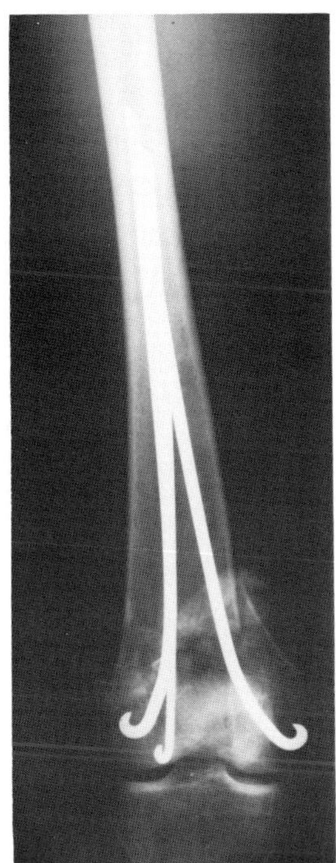

A

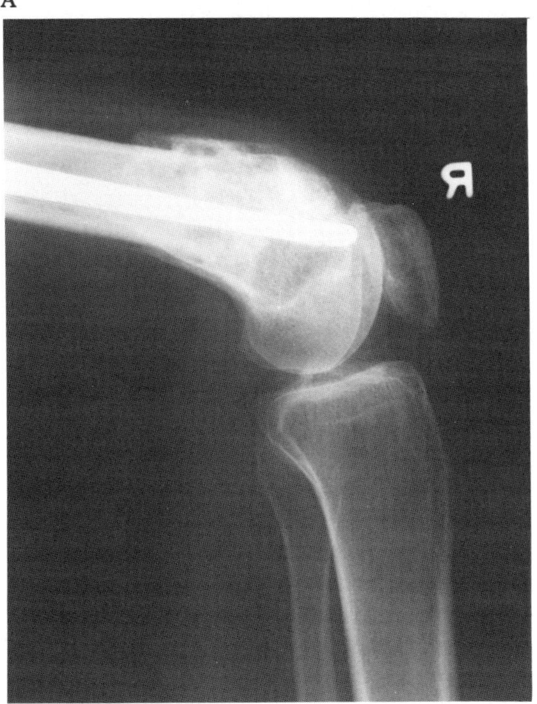

B

Figure 5–46. (**A**) A 17-year-old girl injured in a Halloween automobile accident had an open supracondylar and anteorlateral condylar fracture, as well as a laceration into the right eye orbit. The fracture was reduced on the Rush table with the knee rest. The wounds were debrided and two 3/16-inch (4.76 mm) pins were inserted straight and slightly stress relieved. The anterior condylar fracture was pinned with a straight 1/8-inch (3.18 mm) pin at the edge of the articular surface. At the same time, her right eye was enucleated. (**B**) Part of the comminuted supracondylar fracture was impaled in the quadriceps muscle and 5 months later, after the fracture was healed and motion was still limited, impingement on the quadriceps muscle was released, with removal of the bony fragment, as well as the 1/8-inch (3.18 mm) Rush pin to give good knee motion.

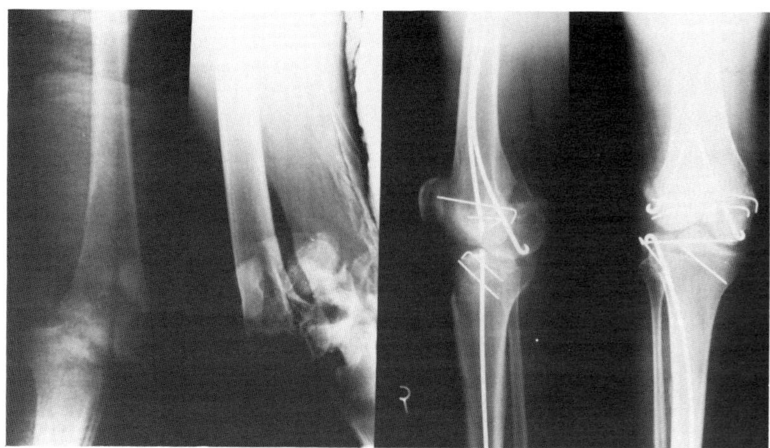

Figure 5–47. An 18-year-old woman with a Gustilo Grade III open fracture, dislocation of the supracondylar and tibila plateau, and a laceration of the patellar tendon was taken to surgery for debridement. The medial femoral condyle was pinned with two Kirschner wires and a ⅛-inch (3.18 mm) Rush pin through the open wounds after debridement. Please see Chapter 13 for further follow-up.

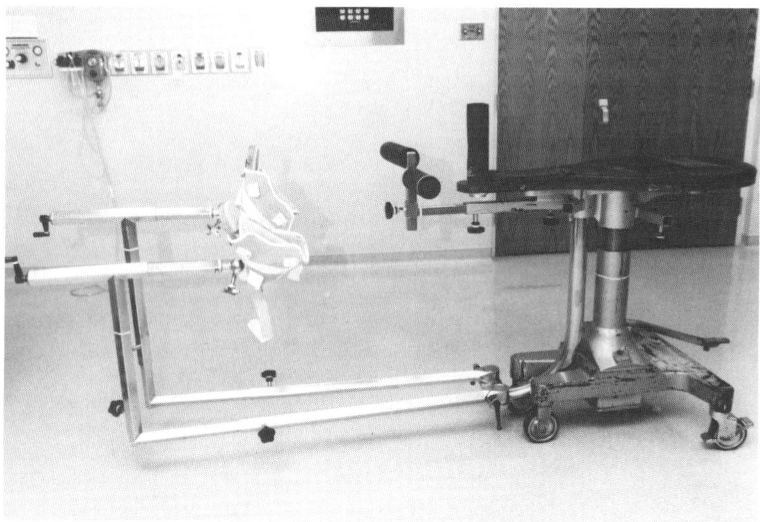

Figure 5–48. The Rush table with the Orthopaedics-Indianapolis offset countersupport is used for bilateral femoral fractures treated at the same time with one image intensifier.

patient is totally asymptomatic and able to bear weight without problems. Early bone grafting is indicated in this situation. One must understand that failure to heal precedes metal failure. Fortunately, the strength of the Rush pin, because of its cold worked stainless-steel condition, keeps metal failure down, but it is still a possibility.

The second pitfall is backing out of the internal fixation device particularly at the knee. This has been remarked on in Chapter 4 and it is related to motion at the fracture site. If this should happen, the pins can have the degree of stress relieving changed by backing the pins out and using a bending iron.

An additional pitfall is the decision to tubulate with cerclage wires to provide stability. The technique of cerclage wiring should be done with minimal dissection of soft tissue, and the areas that are troublesome are those in the distal flare of the femur where the trumpet shape of the femur would allow the wire to slide. In this situation, the soft tissues must be utilized, particularly the linea aspera, which is quite tough and can prevent the wire from migrating. Pinning the joint capsule to the knee or the fascia lata to the hip is always a possibility and will result in painful motion. In the knee, the motion is usually from 0 to approximately 30 degrees and then will be limited by pain.

SUGGESTED READINGS

Clawsen, D.K., Smith, R.F., Hansen, S.T.: Closed intramedullary nailing of the femur, J. Bone Joint Surg. 53A:681–692, 1971.

Eriksson, E., Hovelius, L.: Ender nailing in fractures of diaphysis of the femur. J. Bone Joint Surg. 61A:1175–1181, 1979.

Eriksson, E., Wallin, C.: Immediate or delayed Küntscher-rodding of femoral shaft fractures. Orthopedics 9(2):203, 1986.

Gandolfi, M., Malavolta, L., Tomasso, A.: Dynamic flexible intramedullary nailing in the treatment of fractures of the femoral diaphysis. Ital. J. Orthop. Traumatol. 12(2):159–166, 1986.

Holst-Nielsen, F.: Dynamic intramedullary osteosynthesis in fractures of the femoral shaft. Acta Orthop. Scand. 43:411–420, 1972.

Kempf, I., Grosse, A., Beck, G.: Closed locked intramedullary nailing. Its application to comminuted fractures of the femur. J. Bone Joint Surg. 67A:709–20, 1985.

Leighton, R.K., Waddell, J.P., Kellam, J.P., Orreil, K.G.: Open versus closed medullary nailing of femoral shaft fractures. J. Trauma 26:923–926, 1986.

Maor, P., Pauker, M., Shauer, L., Morein, G.: Closed Rush nailing of femoral fractures. Orthop. Rev. 7(9):91–95, 1978.

Marshall, T.: Closed Rush pin fixation of 235 femoral shaft fractures. Presented at the 71st meeting of the Clinical Orthopaedic Society, Indianapolis, Indiana, October 12, 1983.

Olerud, S., Stromberg, L.: Intramedullary reaming and nailing: its early effects on cortical bone vascularization. Orthopedics 9(9):1204–1208, 1986.

Ong, L.B., Satku, K., Lim, P.H.C.: The treatment of femoral shaft fractures by closed Küntscher nailing (without reaming). Injury 12:466–470, 1980.

Pankovich, A.M.: Adjunctive fixation in flexible intramedullary nailing of femoral fractures. Clin. Orthop. 157:301–309, 1981.

Pankovich, A.M., Goldflies, M.D., Pearson, R.L.: Closed Ender nailing of femoral shaft fractures. J. Bone Joint Surg. 61A:222–232, 1979.

Perry, C.R., Pankovich, S.M., Cohn, S.L.: Locked flexible intramedullary nails in treatment of unstable femoral fractures. J. Orthop. Trauma 1:130–140, 1987.

Rush, L.V.: Atlas of Rush Pin Technics. Meridian, Mississippi, The Berivon Company, 1955.

Rush, L.V., Rush, H.L.: A medullary fracture pin for spring-type fixation: as applied to the femur. Mississippi Doctor September 119–126, 1949.

Shelbourne, D.K., Brueckmann, F.R.: Rush pin fixation of supracondylar and intracondylar fractures of the femur. J. Bone Joint Surg. 64A:161–169, 1982.

Spray, P.: Rush intramedullary nailing of femoral shaft fractures. A possible lifesaver. Contemp. Orthop. 15(2):27–41, 1987.

Tscherene, H., Haas N., Krettek, C.: Intramedullary nailing combined with cerclage wiring in the treatment of fractures of the femoral shaft. Clin. Orthop. 212:62–67, 1986.

Winquist, R.A., Hansen, S.T., Jr., Clawson, D.K.: Closed intramedullary nailing of femoral fractures. J. Bone Joint Surg. 66A:531, 1984.

Fractures of the Tibia

The tibia, because of its weight-bearing importance and subcutaneous location, as well as the frequency of injury, is the bone frequently surgically treated. The shape of the bone at the knee and the shaft and the muscle coverage on three sides present unique problems in the care of the fracture by pin fixation. The problems are:

1. Angulation of the fracture and shortening due to muscle coverage and muscle forces.
2. Angulation and rotation of the fracture due to location of the obliquity of the fracture.
3. Comminution of the fracture.
4. The condition of the fibula.

Reduction of the fracture is essential for planning and execution. The fracture table with countersupport at the knee or a regular table with a countersupport, or even a regular table with the knee maximally bent, will provide support for the knee and allow for reduction of most tibial fractures.

MIDSHAFT FRACTURES

Knee flexion facilitates reduction and insertion of the awl near the medial side of the tibial tuberosity at the proper angle of less than 30 degrees (Fig. 6–1). After the awl is inserted, pin lengths can be determinuted with a rack of ¼-inch (6.35 mm) pins by palpation at the ankle joint. A gentle bend is placed in the pin with a bending iron. The amount of bend varies with the diameter of the medullary canal. The larger the diameter is, the greater the bend should be. The pin is engaged by removing the awl and sliding the tip of the pin in the slot of the awl and exchanging it into the bone. The sled runner is turned to face the opposite cortex after insertion, and when the pin changes direction on impaction, the sound of impaction also changes. When reduction is not perfect (Fig. 6–2A), the pin itself may be used to reduce the fracture. Precurving of the pin, and the sled runner tip, provide a radius equal to or greater than the diameter of the shaft, and manipulation of the head of the pin plus

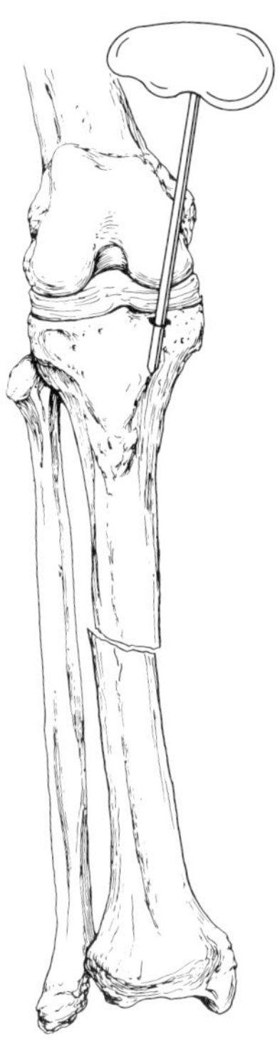

Figure 6–1. Insertion and reduction of fracture by the pin. Fractures of the shaft of the tibia without fractures of the fibula are sometimes difficult to reduce. It is easiest to have the knee bent at least 70 degrees, and this can be done, with some difficulty, on the fracture table. The awl is usually started medial to the patellar tendon. With a standard medullary canal, ¼-inch (6.35 mm) pin is prebent.

impaction can reduce the fracture and immobilize it Fig. 6–2B. After the fracture is reduced, the impacting of the pin with a mallet will have a different sound, and this is indicative of a firmer fixation (Fig. 6–2C).

If reduction is still impossible or is extremely difficult, the semi-open method (Fig. 6-2-D) is used without extra stripping of the periosteum. The stability of the fracture dramatically changes as the pin crosses the fracture.

In seating of the head, the hook should be directed anteriorly and the length and position determined radiographically prior to final impaction.

The Victory Formula

When a pin is inserted in a short fragment to transfix an oblique fracture near the end of the bone (Figs. 6–3, 6–4, and 6–5), if possible, the pin should be directed so that the axis of the shaft of the pin parallels the axis of the fracture. If the pin is put in the opposite direction so that it crosses the fracture line close to right angles, it usually produces displacement of the fracture.

TWO-PIN FIXATION

Fractures in the proximal part of the tibial shaft (Fig. 6–7), tibial plateau fractures, frequently act the same as a femoral supracondylar fracture and will need two-pin stability for fixation. Double ³⁄₁₆-inch (4.76 mm) pins are inserted simultaneously (Fig. 6–8) after positioning the awl on the medial and lateral sides near the anterior portions of the medial collateral ligament and Gerdy's tubercle, with the knee flexed appropriately to be aimed in line with the tibial shaft in the coronal plane. Straight ³⁄₁₆-inch (4.76 mm) pins, 9 to 10 inches (24.13 cm to 26.04 cm) in length, are inserted into the condyle (Fig. 6–9). If the bone is unusually soft, a ³⁄₁₆-inch (4.76 mm) condylar pin may be used. The lateral condyle can be troublesome because of its flare, and the insertion site may need to be moved more anteriorly and medially. The head is directed laterally so that the sled runner engages the opposite cortex. While the pins are driven simultaneously, there is the characteristic feel and sound as the pin bounces off the opposite cortex. If the pin drives too hard, it is probably placed too transversely. If it goes too easily, it may be going out the fracture site. In this event, the direction of the awl should be changed, and if necessary, the tip of the pin can be bent slightly, particularly on the lateral side.

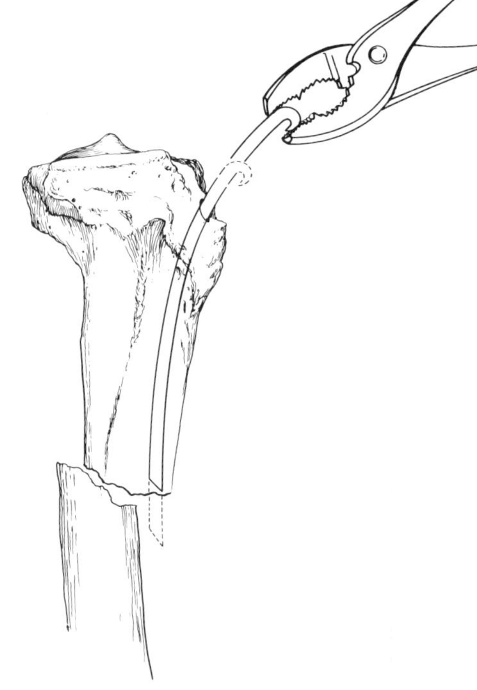

Figure 6–2. (A) A precurved pin misses the fracture site because of incomplete reduction. (B) Pin is backed to the fracture and twisted 180 degrees with the pliers. (C) Impacting the pin across the fracture site is now possible. The pin is twisted back to the original position and then inserted to its full length. The prebent pin is inserted, and the head just grips the awl hole. (D) Reduction of the fracture frequently needs the semi-open technique just to reduce the fracture and allow for passage of the prebent pin across the fracture. The pin is measured from insertion site to the joint line, and then is prebent. If there is concern, the next shorter size is sufficient.

A

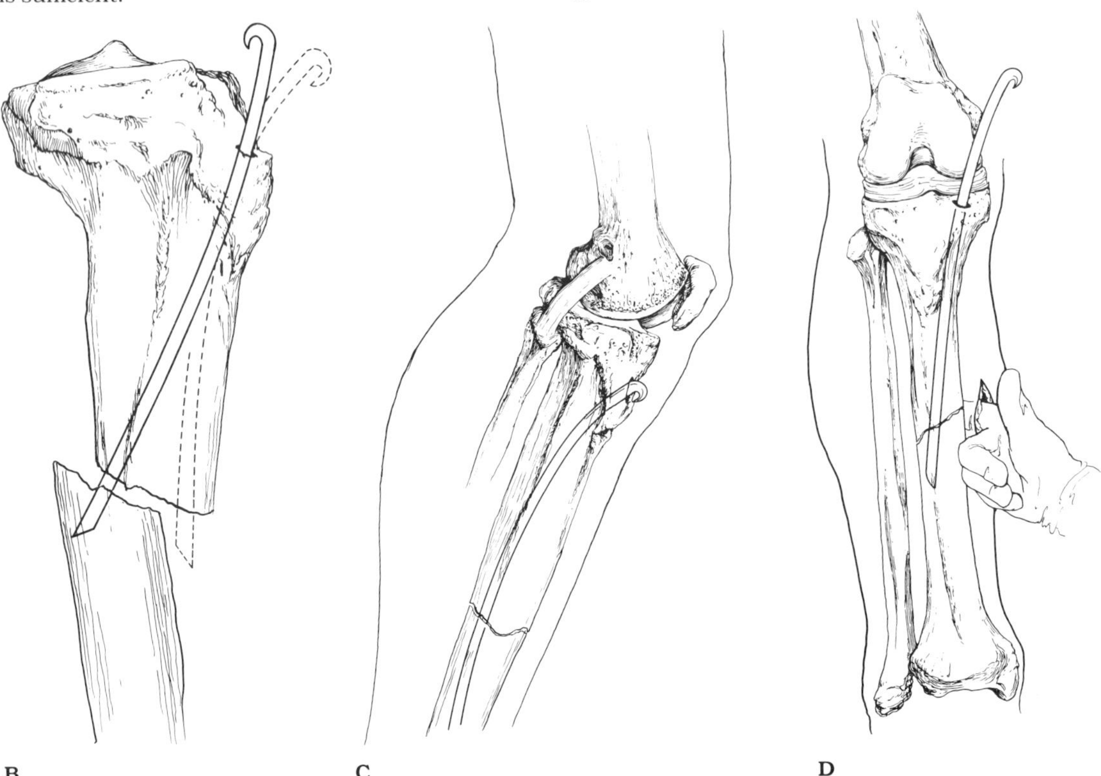

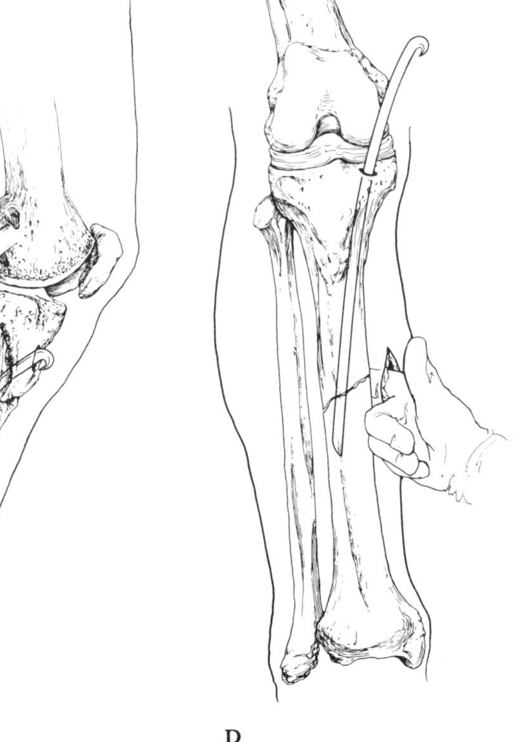

B   C   D

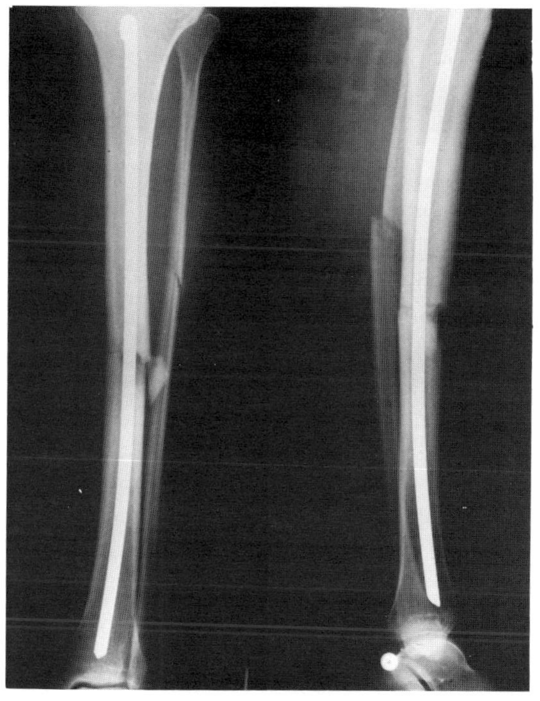
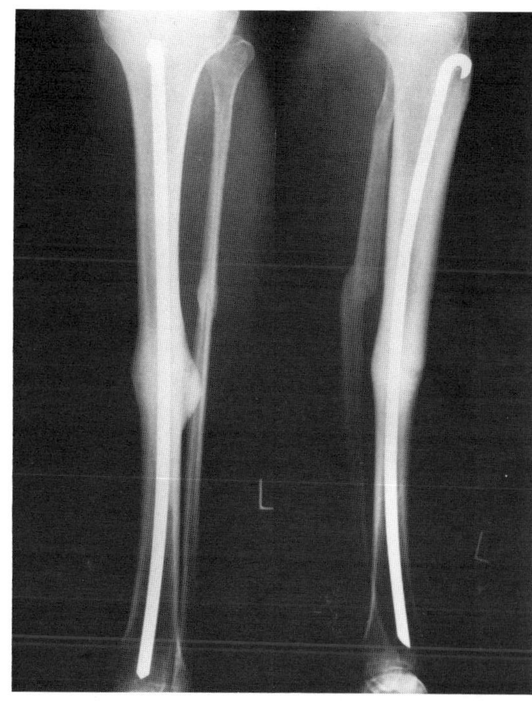

A   B

Figure 6–3.   Closed shaft fracture. (**A**) A 44-year-old female pedestrian who was hit by an automobile at an intersection and thrown on top of the car suffered a closed displaced fracture of the midshaft of the tibia with slight comminution and a fracture of the fibula. Closed pinning with a ¼-inch (6.35 mm) prebent pin within 3 hours after the accident was done. In the following few days the patient was placed in a fabricated brace. Full weight-bearing occurred by the fourth week. (**B**) At 1 year, radiographs showed excellent remodeling of the tibial fracture and incorporation of the loose segment. The patient was scheduled for removal of the ¼-inch (6.35 mm) pin on an outpatient basis.

After the fracture is crossed, the sound of impaction and the stability of the fracture definitely change. The pins may need to be stress relieved somewhat prior to seating unless the bone is very hard.

Comminution of the Tibial Shaft

Comminution frequently needs two ³⁄₁₆-inch (4.76 mm) pins for stability, but these can be inserted more anteriorly and may need to be precured only slightly. Cerclage wiring for long oblique or spiral fractures greatly improves stability. Caution is necessary because the tibia is triangular in shape, and the tip of the wire passer should always be close to the bone so as not to encircle the neurovascular bundles (Fig. 6–10).

Fractures of the Distal End of the Shaft

The single-pin technique will not always stabilize the lower fragment (Fig. 6–11).

The technique just described is excellent for this type of fracture or, as shown, the precurved pin from the lateral condyle can be combined with a similar one driven upward from the lower part of the distal fragment (Fig. 6–12).

Driving a pin upward from the lower

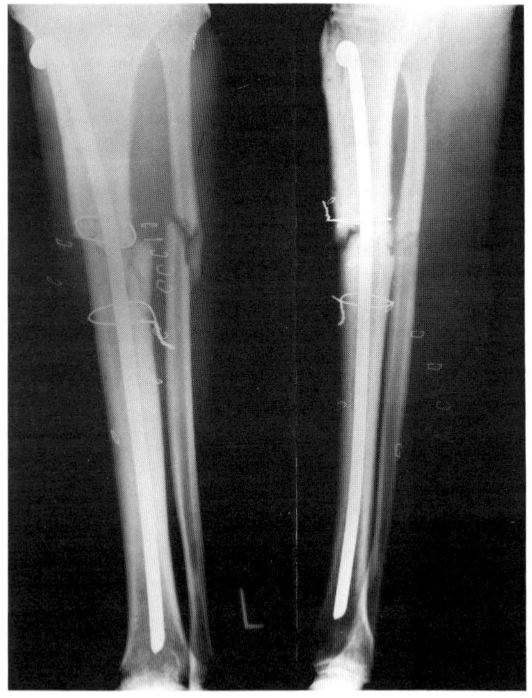
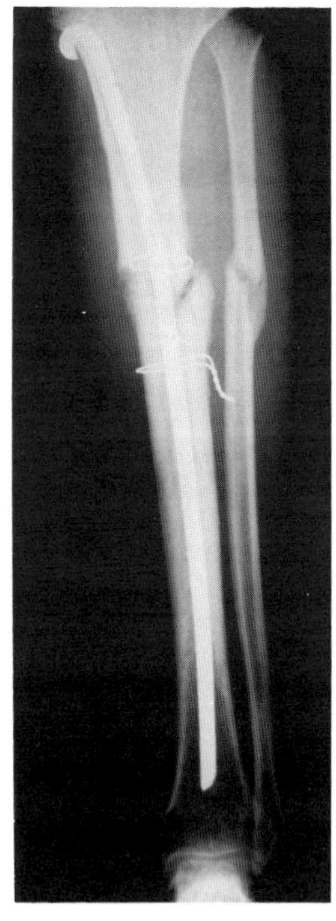
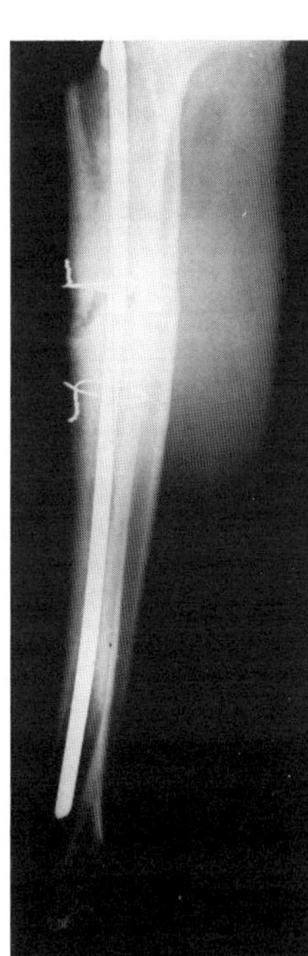

A   B

Figure 6–4.   Open comminuted tibial fracture. (**A**) A 40-year-old motorcyclist had an accident and was unconscious for the first week. He had a Gustilo Grade III tibial fracture that was debrided and about 3 ounces of tibial muscle was removed. Two cerclage wires were used. The fracture was pinned with ¼-inch (6.35 mm) pin, and the wound was left open. Secondary closure was done within a week, and a mesh skin graft was stabled in place. Initial radiographs. (**B**) A cast was put on between the fourth week and the twelfth week and weight-bearing was gradually increased until healing, at 20 weeks without infection. Radiographs at 20 weeks.

fragment can be a frustrating procedure. The opening for the pin should not be in the medial malleolus. It should be proximal and anterior to the medial malleolus and high enough to safeguard against migration of the head of the pin into the joint. A pin that migrates into the ankle is painful and difficult to remove.

If a single straight pin is driven upward through this short lower fragment, angulation will occur unless the proximal portion of the pin is shaped with a bending iron to fit the contour of the bone and, unfortunately, by this procedure, some stability is lost. In this region of the tibia, there is slow healing, and this can be expected. A pin ⅛ inch (3.18 mm) in diameter, in the fibula, will usually provide stability and will help with the healing of the tibia.

Tibial Condyle Fractures

These can be fixed as a closed procedure if reduction can be enhanced by sustaining traction on the fracture table and manipulation. A ³⁄₁₆-inch (4.76 mm) awl is inserted near the joint surface, the awl is used to manipulate the fragment into reduction. While holding it there, another ⅛-inch (3.18 mm) awl can be used to pin the condyle to the center of the plateau and then the ³⁄₁₆-inch (4.76 mm) awl can

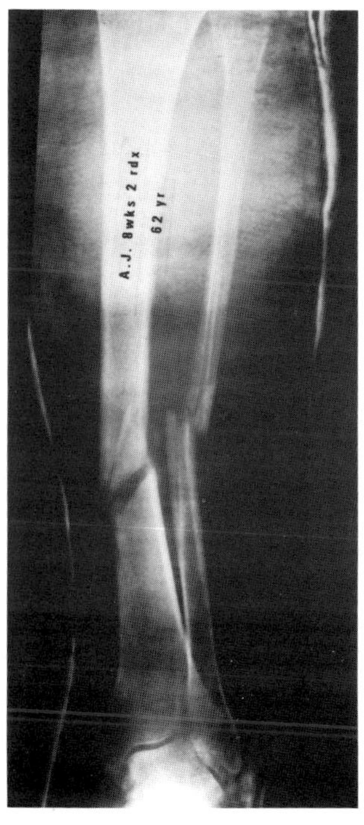
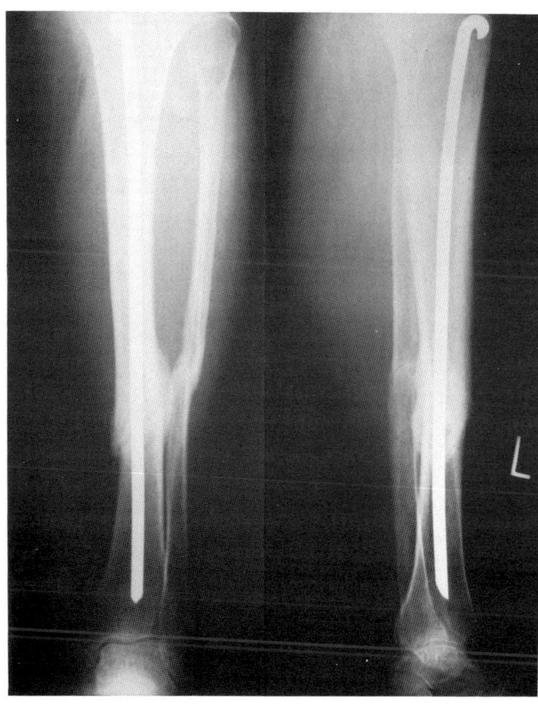

A   B

Figure 6–5.   Delayed fixation and correction of angulation by the pin. (**A**) A 62-year-old woman presented in a long cast 8 weeks, after two manipulations of the tibia under general anesthesia in two separate towns with a resulting valgus deformity still seen on the first radiographs. Closed pinning technique was possible by use of a curved ¼-inch (6.35 mm) pin, with the sled runner tip crossing the fracture line by being twisted with the tip pointed more laterally. After the sled runner crossed the line, the fracture was then straightened and seated. (**B**) A short walking cast was applied for 6 weeks, and the fracture was healed in an additional 6 weeks.

be redirected at the proper angle. A straight ³⁄₁₆-inch (4.76 mm) pin, either regular or looped condylar for soft bone, can be inserted across the fracture site. The resiliency of the pin by the force of impacting the pin against the opposite cortex will provide dynamic compression of the fracture throughout its healing phase.

A "T" or "Y" condylar fracture is done in a similar fashion as supracondylar fractures of the femur. That is, both pins are inserted simultaneously and provide compression of the "T" or the "Y" as the pins are finally seated because of the resiliency of the pins.

SEGMENTAL FRACTURES OF THE TIBIA

It is almost always necessary to use a precurved pin in the treatment of segmental fractures because the reduction of the different segments is so difficult. Manipulation of the pin by manipulating the head of the pin when the pin is curved will allow for reduction of the fracture.

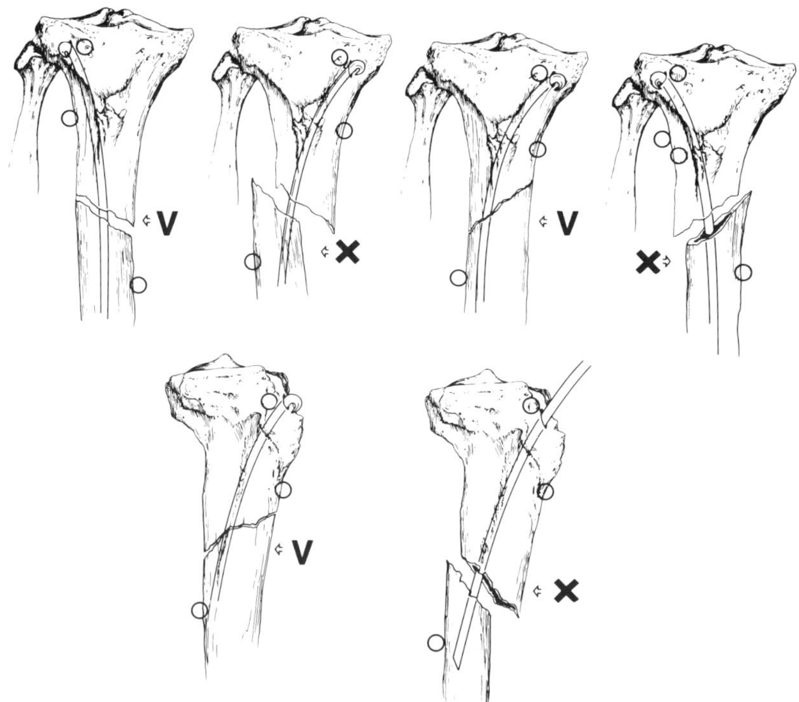

Figure 6–6.   Victory formula. Note the effects of the victory formula, V for closing the fracture and X for distracting the fracture, as mentioned in Chapter 4.

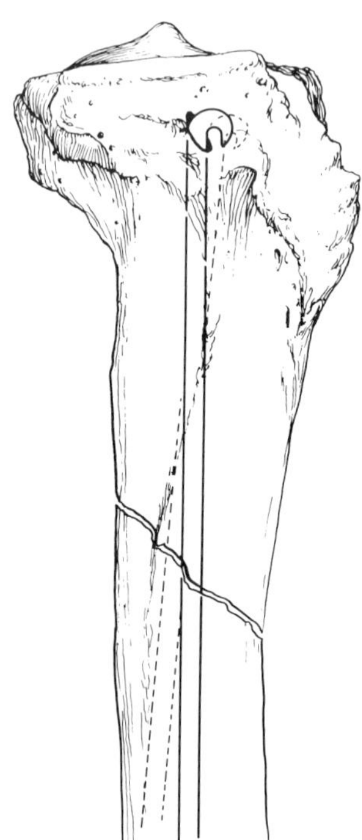

Figure 6–7. An instance in which the victory formula cannot be applied. In this oblique fracture the victory formula cannot be applied. Theoretically, it would be possible to insert the pin from the posterior plateau, but this is not practical. Here it is necessary to use double pins from medial and lateral sides for three-point fixation.

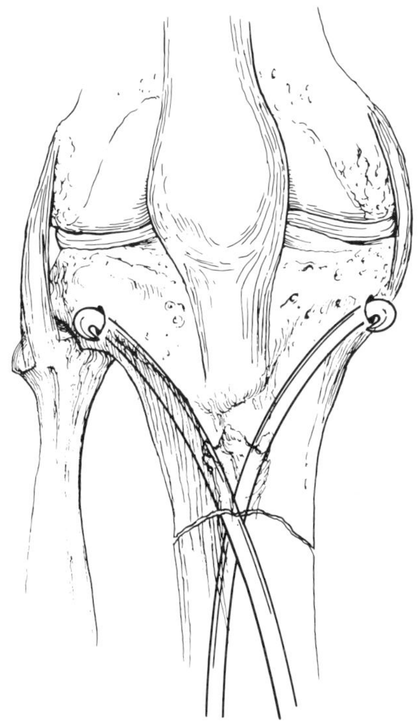

Figure 6–8. Two-pin fixation in the proximal part of the tibia is done percutaneously and is firm enough that early active motion can be started.

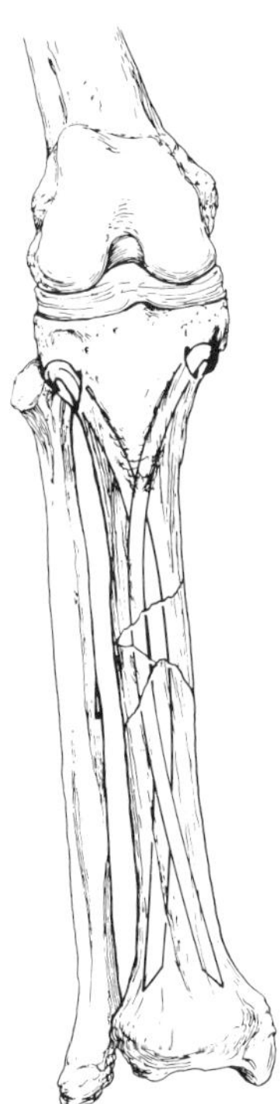

Figure 6–10. Two-pin fixation in comminuted fractures is frequently done. Precurving of the ³⁄₁₆-inch pin is frequently necessary and allows for passage through the comminuted fragments. Occasionally, cerclage wire is practical.

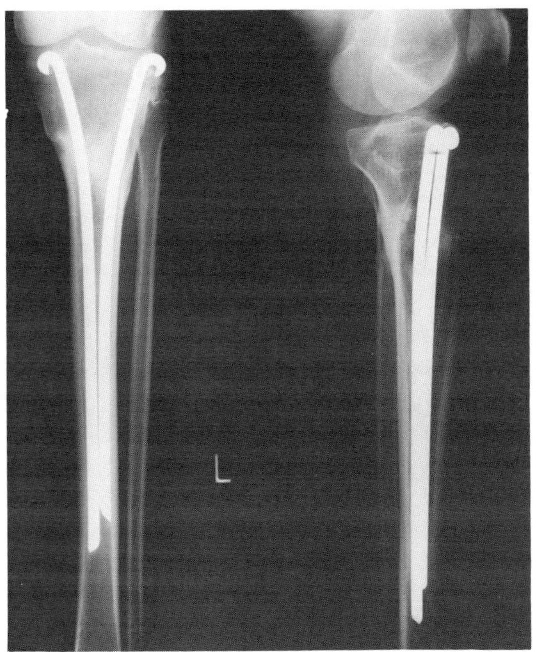

Figure 6–9. A 37-year-old man had a fracture of the proximal part of the tibia and fibula reduced in a closed fashion. Two pins inserted proximally were dynamically bent, similar to the technique for supracondylar fractures.

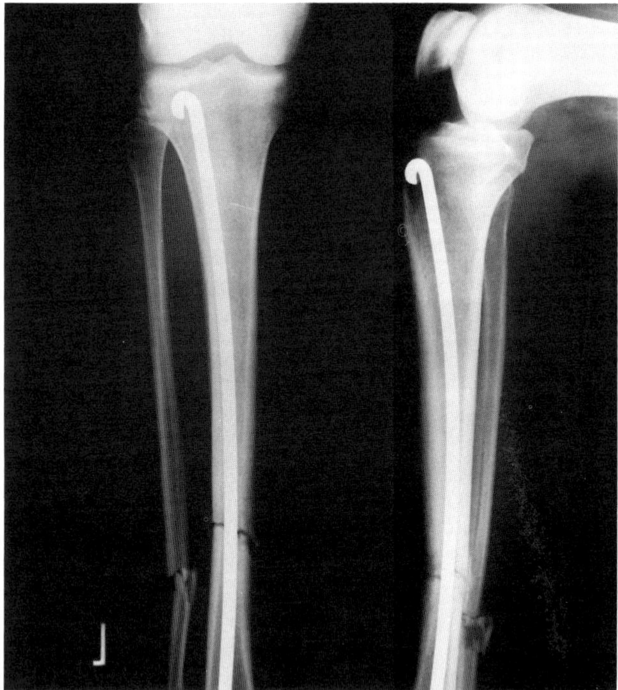

A

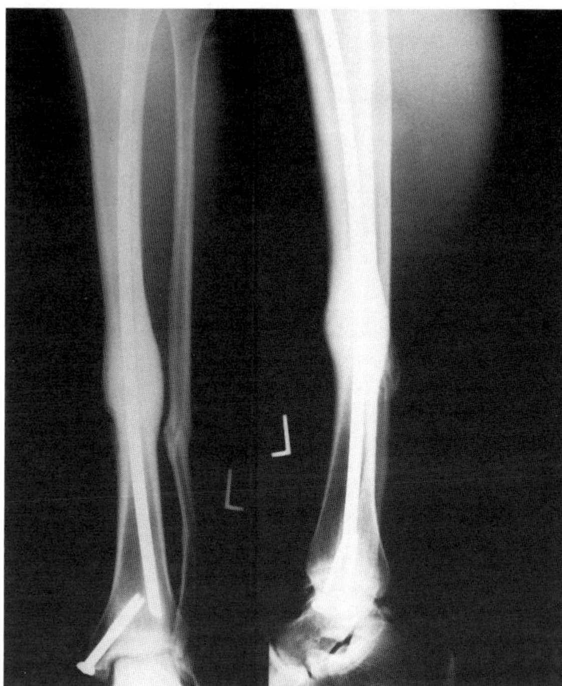

B

Figure 6–11. (**A**) Radiographs of a male with a baseball injury and fracture of the distal part of the tibia and fibula was treated with closed nailing with a curved pin. This gives good stability; a straight pin in the narrow medullary canal would not have given the same degree of stability. (**B**) The radiographs shows healing with abundant callus and remodeling at 9 months. The malleolar screws held the fracture well and motion was initiated early.

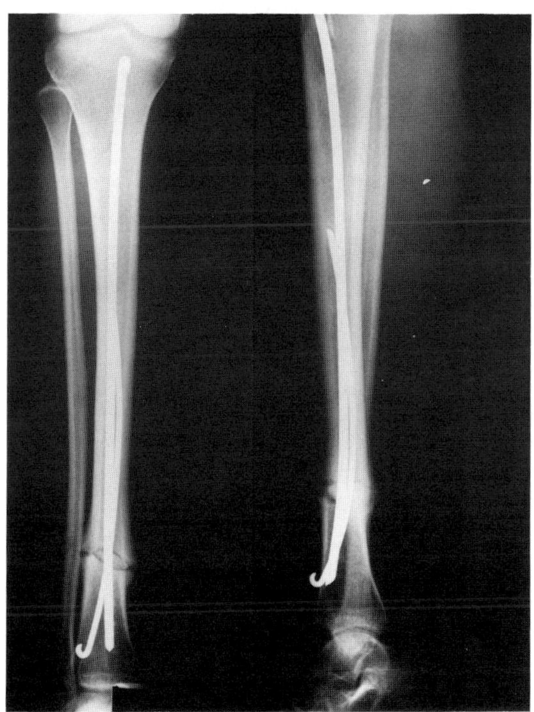

Figure 6–12. A 17-year-old girl was in an auto accident and had a Gustilo Grade II open tibial fracture treated by immediate debridement and two-pin fixation. An attempt was made to use two ³⁄₁₆-inch (4.76 mm) pins, but the medullary canal was too narrow and would not allow the second pin to be seated, so a ⅛-inch (3.18 mm) pin was inserted as demonstrated. Immobilization in a cast was carried out for 3 weeks and weight-bearing initiated when the wound was healed.

SUGGESTED READINGS

Leach, R.E.: A means of stabilizing comminuted distal tibial fractures. J. Trauma 4:722–726, 1964.

Lottes, J.O.: Treatment of delayed or nonunion fractures of the tibia by a medullary nail. Clin. Orthop. 3:111–128, 1965.

Lottes, J.O.: Medullary nailing of the tibia with a tri-flange nail. Clin. Orthop. 105: 253–266, 1974.

Mayer, L., Werbie, T., Schwab, J.P., Johnson, R.P.: The use of Ender's nails in fractures of the tibial shaft. J. Bone Joint Surg. 67A: 446–455, 1985.

Merianos, P., Cambouridis, P., Smyrnis, P.: The treatment of 143 tibial shaft fractures by Ender's nailing and early weight bearing. J. Bone Joint Surg. 67B:576–580, 1985.

Mollica, Q., Gangitano, R., Longo, G.: Elastic intramedullary nailing in shaft fractures of the femur and tibia. Orthopedics 9(8): 1065–1077, 1986.

Rhinelander, F.W.: Minimal internal fixation of tibial fractures. Clin. Orthop. 107:188–220, 1975.

Rush, L.V.: Atlas of Rush Pin Technics. Meridian, Mississippi, The Berivon Company, 1955.

Fractures of the Humerus

It is generally accepted that fractures of the humeral shaft heal rapidly and need surgery infrequently. However, many factors change this dictum, such as:

1. A multiple trauma patient
2. Segmental fractures
3. Bilateral humeral fractures
4. Fractures with arterial involvement
5. Spiral fractures of the distal part of the humerus that may trap the radial nerve (Holstein-Lewis fracture)

With few exceptions, the entire humerus is a beautiful field for medullary pinning. Semi-open reduction is the general rule. In fresh fractures, it is rarely necessary to endanger nerves or impair blood supply of the bone by wide dissection.

FRACTURES OF THE PROXIMAL PART OF THE HUMERUS

The proximal end of the humoral shaft offers definite problems. Atrophy of the deltoid and periarticular adhesions of the shoulder occur very rapidly if function of the shoulder is arrested. Proper utilization of the dynamic forces at different levels of the shaft is essential if nonunion is to be avoided. The important factors are distraction, tendency to angulation, and rotary stresses. They are most conspicuous at the level just distal to the insertion of the deltoid.

ANATOMY

Topographic anatomy is important, and the bicipital groove by palpation is normally in the same position as the bicipital tendon at the elbow in the anteroposterior plane. The acromion, with its attachment to the deltoid, does not completely overhang the humerus, leaving the rotator cuff still palpable. Care must be taken to avoid placement of the pin through the attachment of the rotator cuff to the greater tuberosity, as this will restrict shoulder motion. The superolateral portion and surface of the greater tuberosity, lateral to the bicipital groove and distal to the rotator cuff, are ideal for insertion of a ¼-inch (6.35 mm) or a ³⁄₁₆-inch (4.76 mm) pin, as there is no muscular attachment there, and the axillary nerve and posterior humeral circumflex artery are relatively far away. Distally the radial nerve winds posteriorly about the shaft and can be injured by long spiral fractures in this area. The nerve is proximal to the olecranon fossa on the posterior aspect, which allows a safe entrance for retrograde insertion of Rush pins for shaft fractures.

The epicondyles of the humerus are flat and quite narrow in the medullary canal. Closed reduction of supracondylar fractures of the humerus almost always need the use of an image intensifier to guide the awl through the narrow marrow cavity to get to the fracture site. In older people a wide canal makes this approach easier.

Intramedullary use of the Rush pin is greatly aided by the semi-open technique: (1) finding the fracture site; (2) image intensification; (3) or both. The diameter of the pin will vary from ¼-inch (6.35 mm) to ⅛-inch (3.18 mm), depending on the size of the medullary canal and the location of the fracture.

INSERTION SITES

Proximally

The area lateral, anterior, and inferior to the rotator cuff is ideal for an approach to the neck as well as the shaft of the humerus.

Distally

There are two condyles of the humerus at the elbow and an area of the humerus proximal to the olecranon fossa on the posterior aspect of the humerus that are easily accessible for entrance sites of Rush pins.

Because of the difficulty in placing a humerus in a traction situation, the semi-open technique is frequently easiest, as it allows for better reduction of the fracture by manipulation and palpation with the finger and for easier direction of the awl by aiming at the finger in the wound.

The image intensifier can be used for reduction and observation of the proper position of awl insertion and with skill, the semi-open technique can be avoided. For insertion in the distal end of the humerus, two areas can be used: the medial and lateral condyles, and the posterior part of the humerus, proximal to the olecranon fossa. The condylar approach is used for supracondylar fractures and fractures of the distal end of the shaft. Care must be taken to avoid the ulnar nerve. The medullary canal at the condyles is difficult to get into in young people, and less of a problem in the elderly; it usually will accept a ⅛-inch (3.18 mm) pin.

The area proximal to the olecranon

fossa is approached through a VanGorder splitting incision in the triceps. Cortical bone is difficult to penetrate with an awl, so a drill or a burr is used to develop an oblique window into the medullary canal. This has been described by Hackethal[1] and later by Durbin et al.[2] and Pritchett.[3]

SHAFT FRACTURES

The operation is done as a semi-open procedure with the arm draped so that it can be manipulated, or the operation can be done with a closed technique using an image intensifier with the person in the supine position (Fig. 7–1). A small incision is made at the level of the fracture. The anterolateral surface is usually used.

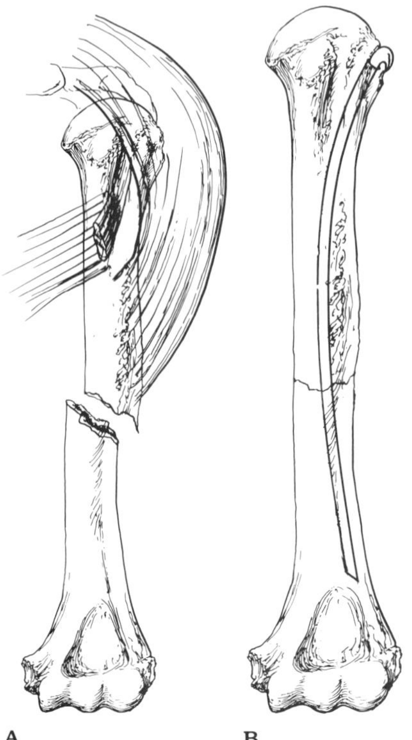

Figure 7–1. Shaft fractures. **(A)** Shaft fractures are easily treated by the semi-open method with the awl directed toward the finger at the fracture. **(B)** A precurved pin is put across the fracture site and is short enough so that it does not distract the fracture.

The fascia is split, and the fracture is palpated with a finger. The awl is passed through the fibers of the deltoideus at the neutral area to engage the cortex of the surgical neck of the humerus, distal to the rotator cuff. After the cortex has been penetrated, the awl is gradually changed to an angle of 20 to 30 degrees to the long axis of the humerus. It is at this time that palpation of the fracture site with the opposite hand is quite helpful.

The pin, preferably ¼-inch (6.35 mm) in diameter and slightly curved, or ³⁄₁₆-inch (4.76 mm) in diameter and slightly curved, is driven to the fracture line after exchanging it with the awl in the proximal part of the humerus (Fig. 7–2). After reduction is palpated, the pin is then driven into the distal fragment, being careful that the pin does not cause distraction by hitting the bone supporting the olecranon fossa.

The head of the pin should be slightly stress relieved and left somewhat prominent for easy removal. Fractures above insertion of the deltoid are enveloped in a strong muscular envelope and usually heal readily. Fractures below the insertion are frequently fraught with nonunion, and pin placement is extremely important. The deltoid tends to pull the proximal fragment laterally, and the fractures are usually oblique. As with fractures of the shaft of the tibia, when the obliquity of the fracture and the angle of the pin form a V, the fracture is usually stable; in those fractures in which the obliquity is the opposite, the fractures usually shorten and nonunion is frequent. The use of ¼-inch (6.35 mm) or ³⁄₁₆-inch (4.76 mm) precurved pins is essential. If the obliquity is such that displacement would be possible, the insertion site should be moved just adjacent to the long head of the biceps tendon, and the pin placed in a more anteroposterior plane, being very careful not to have the pin so long that it engages the area of the olecranon fossa and causes distraction (Fig. 7–3). Another solution

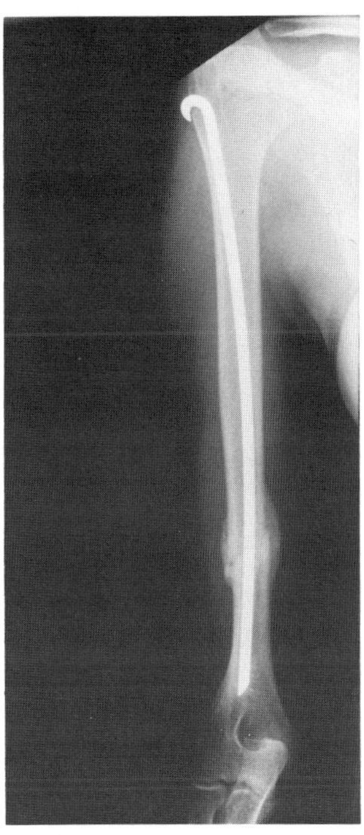

Figure 7–2. A 22-year-old victim of an automobile accident had bilateral femoral shaft fractures (Gustilo Grade II on the right side), fracture of the distal end of the right tibial shaft, fracture of the right humerus, concussion, and severe facial injuries on May 27, 1988. Same day surgery was performed using the fracture table with the bilateral knee countersupport where both femurs were pinned, one from the greater trochanter and one from the lateral condyle, with cerclage wires. At the same time, closed pinning of the tibia was done in the same surgical prepping by two surgeons. After this, the right humerus was pinned using a closed technique and the image intensifier. At the first office visit, after 4 weeks of hospitalization, on the June 22, 1988, the humerus was healed and the patient was using the arm for getting in and out of a wheelchair. Additional radiographs are shown in Chapter 12.

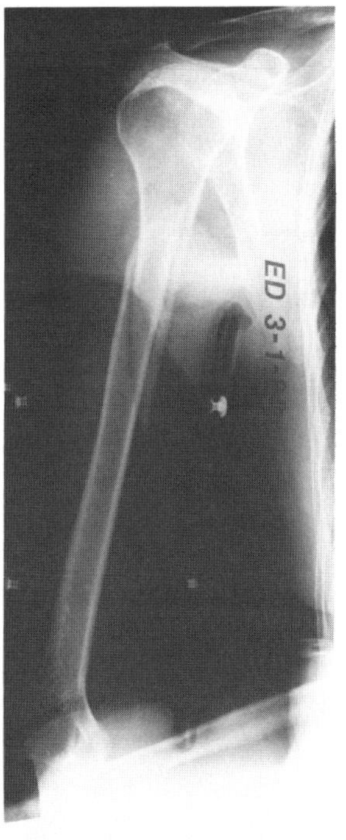

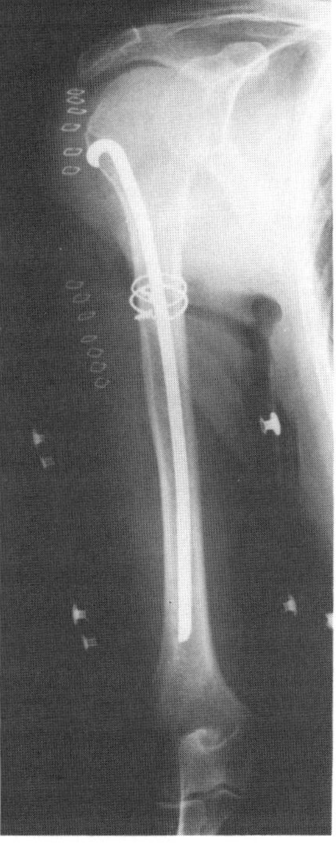

Figure 7–3. Fracture of the proximal end of the shaft (**A**) A 75-year-old female diabetic taking insulin had a displaced humeral fracture on the right side and a Colles' fracture on the left. (**B**) Early mobilization so that the right hand could be used was done with pin fixation and minimal exposure for cerclage wire and insertion of a ³⁄₁₆-inch (4.76 mm) prebent pin. Early functional use was started with a plastic arm sleeve.

A   B

for this problem fracture is to do multiple pinning from distal supraolecranon fossa area as described by Hackethal.[1] In this position, the cortical window is made on the posterior aspect of the humerus, proximal to the olecranon fossa, and is enlarged so that it is close to 1 cm (⅖ inch) in diameter and at an angle to provide access to the humerus. Multiple ⅛-inch (3.18 mm) precurved pins of an appropriate length are used. The number is dependent on the size of the entrance window as filling the window provides part of the three-point fixation for the pin.

Again, the basic principles for using a curved pin in a straight bone or a straight pin in a curved bone apply. That is, precurved pins should be used for the shaft, and straight pins should be inserted dynamically from the side for fractures in the proximal or distal ends.

FRACTURES OF THE HUMERAL NECK

Closed Pinning

Closed pinning is often indicated in the elderly (Fig. 7–4). It can be very simple or very difficult. Displacement is when the upper fragment is pulled outward by the supraspinatus and the pectoralis major pulls the shaft medially. This is continuous and can cause delayed deformity if the fracture is not pinned.

Technique

The fracture should be reduced and a ³⁄₁₆-inch (4.76 mm) pin used. If the bone is osteoporotic, the loop condylar pin or two ⅛-inch (3.18 mm) pins can be used. The sled runner point is directed toward the far cortex to guide it down the shaft. The pin is set, and the stab wound is closed. A sling is used for immobilization. The pin

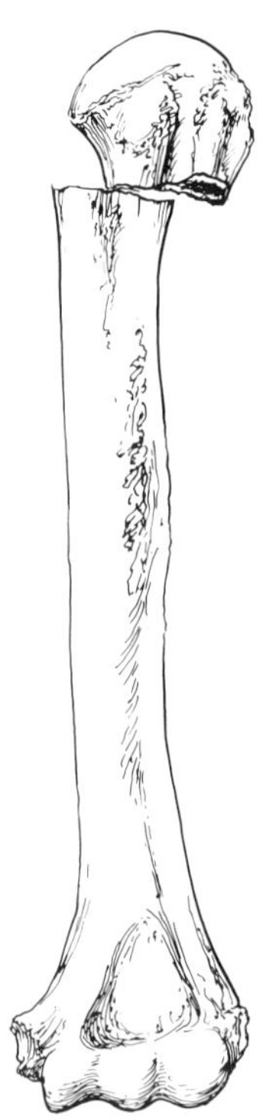

Figure 7–4.   Transverse neck fractures. The pectoralis major pulls the shaft medially. A ⅛-inch (3.18 mm) or ³⁄₁₆-inch (4.76 mm) pin placed outside the rotator cuff resists this pull by exerting three-point pressure. This is frequently done as a closed procedure, but if there is a question, the semi-open technique is quite acceptable.

exerts three-point pressure in the bone and resists muscle pull.

When closed pinning is not practical, a small anterior incision is made and the semi-open technique is used for reduction of the fracture (Fig. 7–5). Insertion of the awl in a neutral area and the use of a ³⁄₁₆-inch (4.76 mm) or multiple ⅛-inch (3.18 mm) pins is helpful.

SUPRACONDYLAR FRACTURES

The technique for fixation of supracondylar fractures is but a modification of that used in the supracondylar fracture of the femur, with which one should be thoroughly familiar before embarking on a

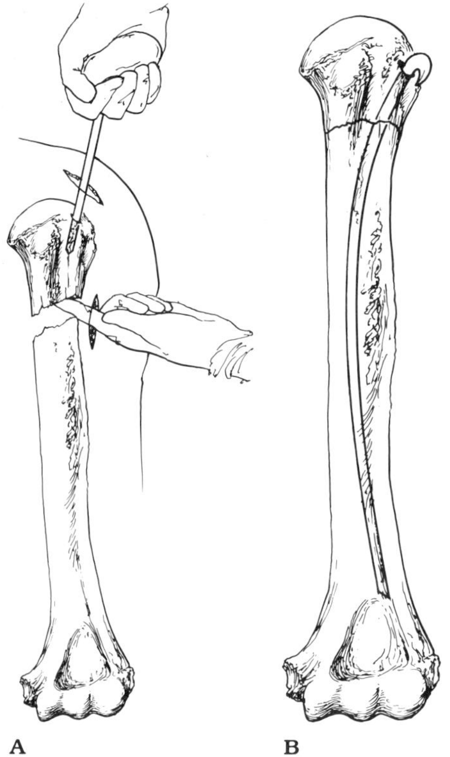

A   **B**

Figure 7–5. Semi-open technique for neck fractures. **(A)** The pin is introduced through a stab incision outside of the rotator cuff, with the awl aimed toward the palpating finger at the fracture site. The grooved awl is used to direct the pin into the hole an the pin is impacted into place. This is a much more simple technique, as it is difficult to get satisfactory image intensification views in this area. **(B)** Position of curved pin in humerus with a neck fracture.

similar procedure in the elbow (Fig. 7–6). The elbow region is much more complex. Great stability can be obtained by dynamic fixation with ⅛-inch (3.18 mm) straight pins inserted across the fracture and developing a bend from the angle of insertion. The three-point fixation provides stability. The VanGorder approach is safe but muscle stripping should be avoided as much as possible. Cerclage wires can be used, with the same admonition.

Technique

The fracture is reduced by open reduction, and the fragments are held in posi-

tion manually. The pins are ⅛-inch (3.18 mm) in diameter and of sufficient length to extend well into the medullary canal of the shaft of the humerus. With the awl reamer, and care being taken to avoid the ulnar nerve, insertion sites are placed in the medial and lateral epicondyles, with the pins directed toward the center of the shaft. The pins are exchanged for the awl and driven simultaneously so that the sled runners bounce off the cortex of the intramedullary canal, develop a bend in the pin, and provide dynamic fixation (Fig. 7–7). At close to final insertion, it is frequently necessary to bend the remaining portion of the pins with the bending iron, to stress relieve it and confirm with the contour of the distal end of the humerus in order to avoid migration of the heads of the pins into the bone. The heads should be left prominent but should not engage the capsule (Figs. 7–8, 7–9).

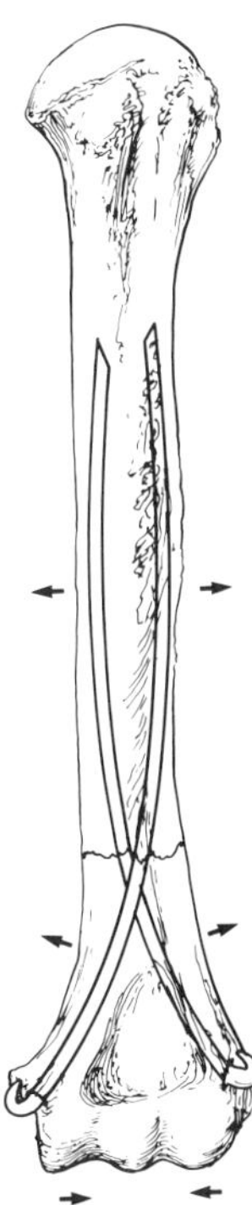

Figure 7–6. Supracondylar fracture. Long pins that are bent by impaction provide three-point fixation.

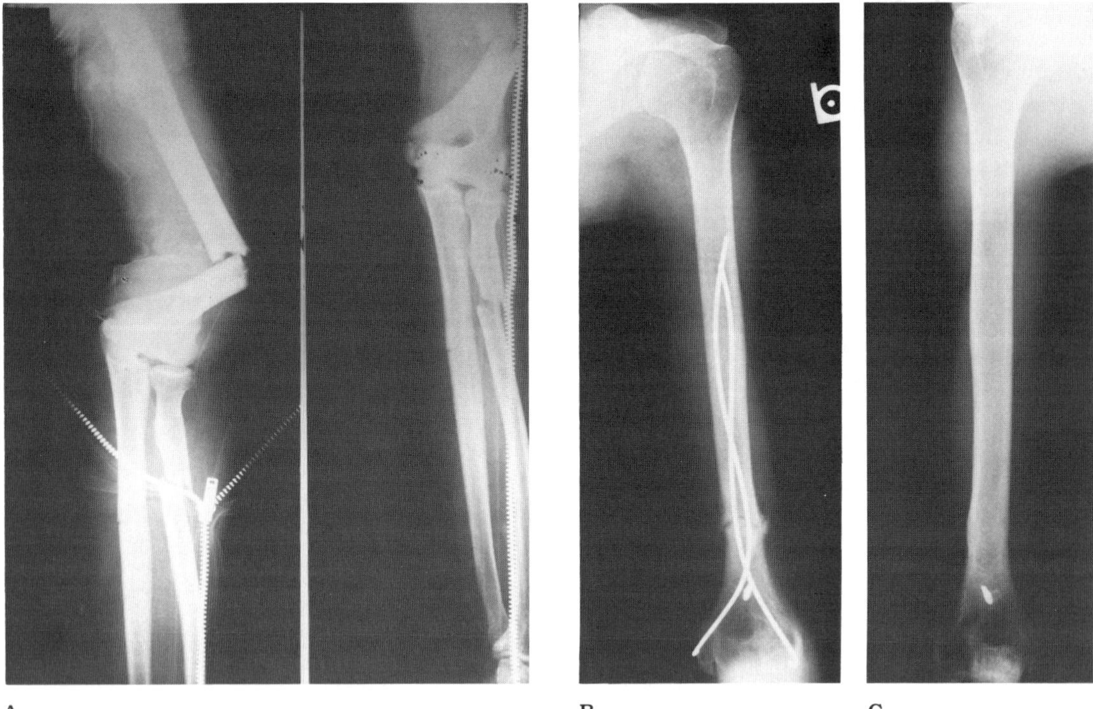

A   B   C

Figure 7–7.   (A) A 34-year-old male motorcyclist had a segmental fracture of the distal part of the humeral shaft and a moderately undisplaced supracondylar fracture below it, along with a fracture of the proximal parts of the radius and ulna. (B) In April 1974, he was treated with two ³⁄₃₂-inch (2.38 mm) Rush pins going across the supracondylar fracture, as well as the segmental transverse humeral fracture. (C) Pins were removed 13 months after the time of fracture, and the bone showed little evidence of "fracture disease."

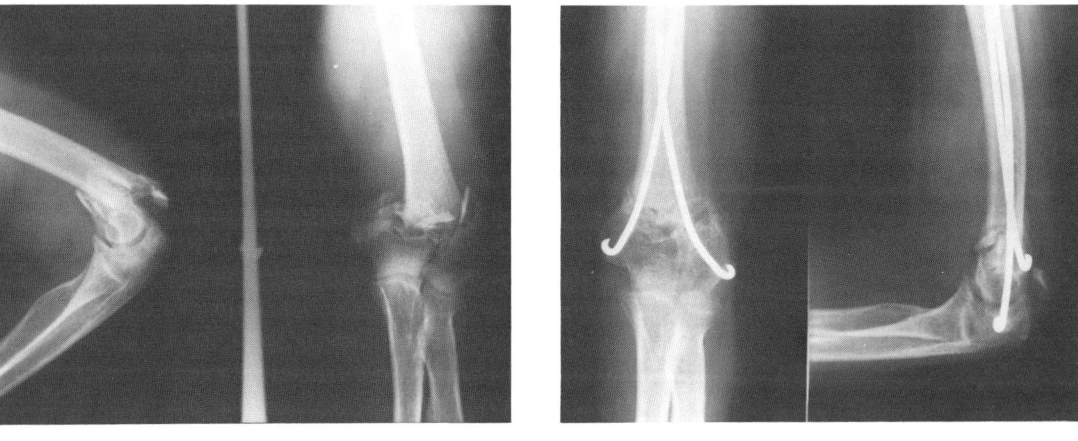

A   B

Figure 7–8.   (A) A 54-year-old woman had a displaced intracondylar and supracondylar fracture of the humerus treated with closed pinning with two ⅛-inch (3.18 mm) straight pins. She was able to function early. (B) Radiographs were made at 6 weeks postoperatively in September 1972 (continued).

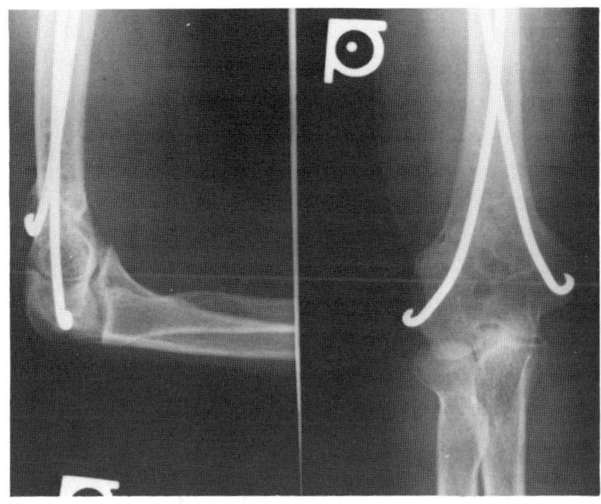

C

Figure 7–8 (cont.). (C) At routine follow-up in April 1974, complete healing and remodeling were noted, with a range of motion from 20 to 120 degrees.

Comminuted osteoporotic fractures of the neck with marked medial displacement of the distal fragment due to pull by the pectoralis major may be salvaged by percutaneously pinning the humerus in the following manner. A ¼-inch (6.35

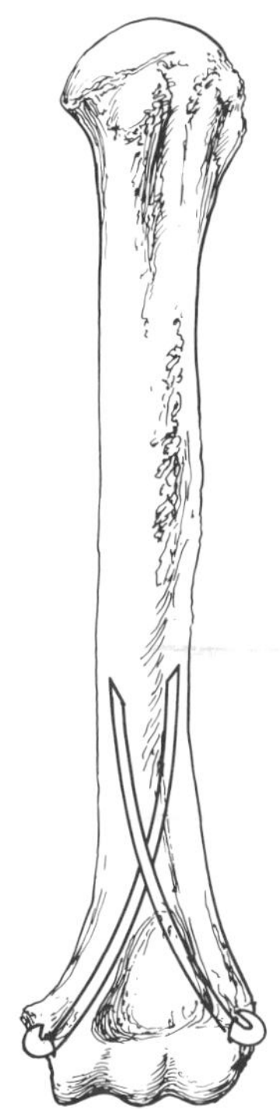

Figure 7–9. Pins should be impacted to the cortex and not engage the capsule.

mm) awl hole is placed in the acromion slightly posterior to the acromioclavicular joint and a ³⁄₁₆-inch (4.76 mm) pin is then placed across the acromion through the rotator cuff, through the head, and into the shaft. This will provide stability. The pin is usually bent at right angles in the last inch so that it will not slide down into the hole and disappear into the humerus. Pin removal is possible after 3 to 4 weeks of immobilization in a sling and swathe, and surprising function often results in the osteoporotic patient.

POSTOPERATIVE MANAGEMENT

Prevention of joint ankylosis and continued fracture coaptation in the shaft are the primary problems. Active and passive range-of-motion exercises are beneficial for fractures of the proximal and distal ends of the humerus. Frequently a sugar tong cast applied in the area of the supracondylar fracture, to control swelling and allow some motion, is helpful. Exercises to prevent distraction can be done in the alert patient, by asking the patient to attempt to squeeze the elbow into the flank and chest, first on the normal side and then on the fractured side. This maneuver inevitably causes the biceps and triceps to contract and compress the fracture.

Joint stiffness, particularly in the osteoporotic bone, is a prerunner to slow healing and disability with a fracture. Attention must be paid to joint immobilization.

REFERENCES

1. Hackethal, K.H.: Die Bundel-Nagelung. Berlin, Springer, 1961, p 134.
2. Durbin, R.A., Gottesman, M.J., Sanders, K.C.: Hackethal stacked nailing of humeral shaft fractures. Clin. Orthop. 179:168–174, 1983.
3. Pritchett, J.W.: Delayed union of humeral shaft fractures treated by closed flexible intramedullary nailing. J. Bone Joint Surg. 67:715–718, 1985.

SUGGESTED READINGS

Grimes, D.W.: The use of Rush pin fixation in unstable upper humeral fractures. Orthop. Rev. 9:75–79, 1980.
Hall, R.F., Pancovich, A.M.: Technique and results of closed flexible intramedullary rodding of diaphyseal fractures of the humerus. Orthop. Trans. 6:359, 1982.
Holstein, A., Lewis, G.B.: Fractures of the humerus with radial nerve paralysis. J. Bone Joint Surg. 45A:1382–1388, 1963.
Rush, L.V.: Atlas of Rush Pin Technics. Meridian, Mississippi, The Berivon Company, 1955.
Rush, L.V., Rush, H.L.: Intramedullary fixation of fractures of the humerus by the longitudinal pin. Surgery 27(2):268–275, 1950.
Stern, P.J., Mattingly, D.A., Pomeroy, D.L., et al.: Intramedullary fixation of humeral shaft fractures. J. Bone Joint Surg. 66A:639–646, 1984.

Fractures of the Radius and Ulna

In 1936, Katie Bell Remhert presented to the Doctors Rush with a comminuted Monteggia fracture of the elbow. They used an intramedullary Steinmann pin and cerclage wires for fixation of the fracture. This was reported in 1937.[1] Since that time, the pin technique used currently was developed with experience and experimentation.

MONTEGGIA FRACTURE

The Monteggia fracture precipitated the old Burma Shave road sign slogan: "Elbows held out of the window far, often go home in another car." For fixation a straight ⅛-inch (3.18 mm) pin is inserted from the side of the olecranon into the distal part of the ulna, with cerclage wires placed extraperiosteally on the anterior aspect of the ulna and tightened until the bone is tubulated before the pin is finally inserted. A pin of sufficient length will extend almost to within 2 cm of the styloid process of the ulna. Occasionally the radial head is unstable and needs to be reduced, the annular ligament repaired, and instability discerned (Fig. 8–1). If the Monteggia fracture does not have a specific fracture of the ulna into the articular surface, the awl reamer is

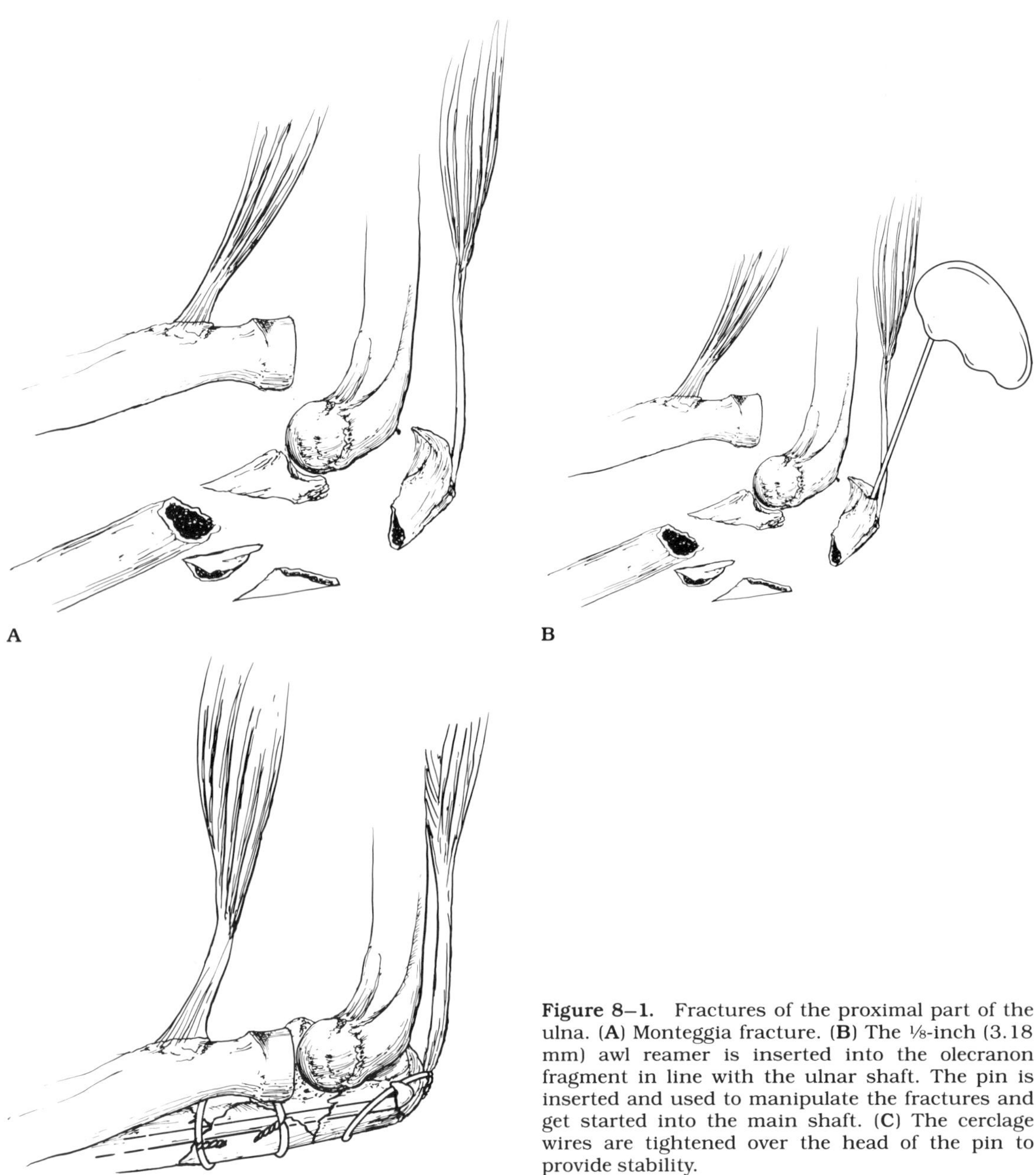

Figure 8–1.   Fractures of the proximal part of the ulna. **(A)** Monteggia fracture. **(B)** The ⅛-inch (3.18 mm) awl reamer is inserted into the olecranon fragment in line with the ulnar shaft. The pin is inserted and used to manipulate the fractures and get started into the main shaft. **(C)** The cerclage wires are tightened over the head of the pin to provide stability.

inserted into the radial side of the olecranon with great care to miss the articular surface. The pin is then passed through the fracture site and impacted into the medullary canal of the shaft. Even if the head of the radius is unstable,

it should be reduced at this time, and then cerclage wires tightened. The pin is continued to be impacted at this time. As the sled runner goes down the medullary canal of the ulna, the head of the pin will curve from side to side. Final seating is done with an impactor. If at this time the radial head is unstable in pronation and supination, the joint can be stabilized with a ⅛-inch (3.18 mm) pin going across the radial humeral joint into the proximal part of the radius, and left subcutaneously in the posterior triceps so that it can be removed at a later date. Unfortunately, this slows down function of the elbow and should be avoided if at all possible. If the pin is left across the joint for too many weeks, the pin may fracture at the joint. The broken pin may be left if it doesn't interfere with joint function. Leaving the pin prominent can allow removal without difficulty.

FRACTURE OF THE OLECRANON

Fracture of the olecranon is treated by intramedullary fixation with a tension band wire technique and has proved to be quite satisfactory. Single-pin fixation is usually not stable enough. Usually two ⅛-inch (3.18 mm) awls are inserted from the sides of the olecranon by splitting the triceps tendon expanse and aiming the awl at 30 degrees to the long axis of the ulna (Fig. 8–2). The patient is usually positioned supine, with a pad placed under the shoulder and the arm across the chest. In fractures with marked displacement, the awl may be retrograded and the pin placed across the fracture, allowing the pin to help with the reduction and the use of the awl on the opposite side. The proximal part of the ulna is quite curved, with a distinct radial bow. Thus, pins placed on the lateral side of the ulna at the proper angle will look as if they parallel the long axis of the forearm. If the awl reamer is inserted at 30 degrees to the long axis of the forearm, the sled runner may penetrate the medial aspect of the ulna and the pin may go into the flexor muscle mass (Fig. 8–3). Occasionally two ³⁄₃₂-inch (2.38 mm) Rush pins are needed because of the narrow canal,

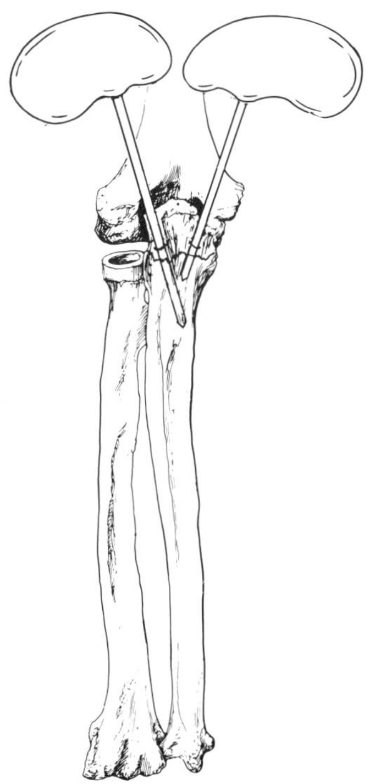

Figure 8–2. The direction of the awl must compensate for the curve in the proximal part of the ulna or the pins will come out of the medullary canal when impacted.

but pins only need to be 4 to 5 inches (10 to 12.5 cm) in length. The tension band wire is inserted through a hole, started on the medial aspect of the ulna to avoid the ulnar nerve. The wire is then crossed in a figure eight fashion and placed over the hooks of the Rush pins, which are turned so that they will hold the wire (Fig. 8–4). The tension band is then tightened and the pins are inserted; this should provide stability. A soft bandage and early motion are the key to a good result. Comminuted fractures with the triceps fascia attached to the fragments will usually stay in place with this technique and will heal with active motion.

The olecranon technique with the tension band wire is frequently used for a Monteggia fracture with the fracture line going into the olecranon fossa.

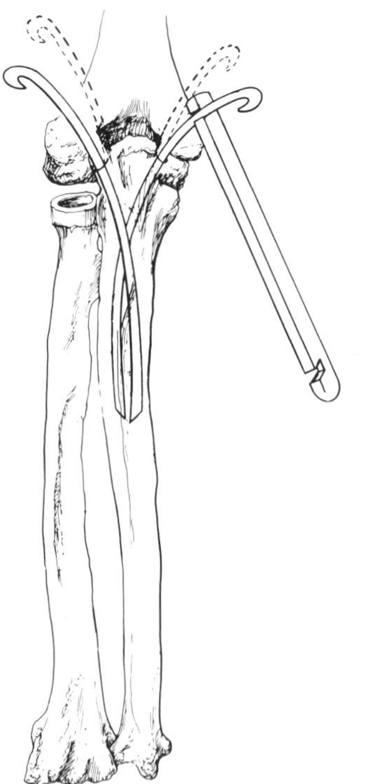

Figure 8–3.   Stress relieving may be needed if the bone is soft.

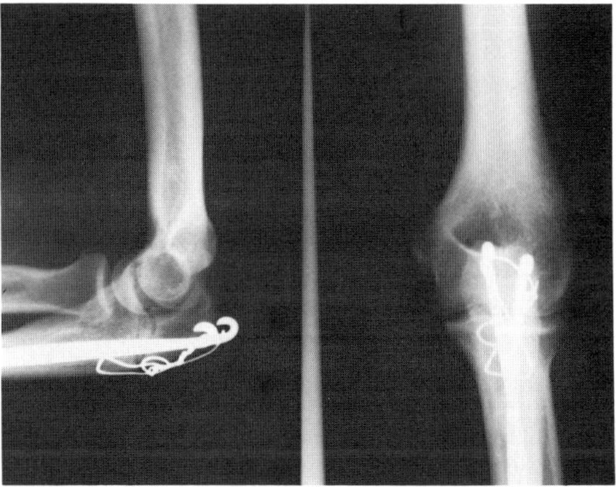

Figure 8–4.   Tension band wires are looped over the head of the pins, which are then impacted.

MEDULLARY PINNING OF FRACTURES IN THE FOREARM

History

Sage,[2] in 1959, used a nail inserted after open reaming in both directions of the medullary canal of the ulna and radius. This technique resulted in a nonunion rate of 12 percent. Caden,[3] in 1961, used Rush pins with a retrograde open technique, with poor results in the radius and ulna. Aho[4] reported the cases of 50 patients who were treated between 1966 and 1977. Forty had fractures of both bones of the forearm, and 39 were treated by closed pinning. Casts were worn for 9 weeks. Ninety percent of the fractures healed in 4 months; one was treated with a bone graft at that time so that eventually 100 percent of the fractures healed. The rate of infection was 0. After removal of the implant no fractures were noted when load-sharing Rush pins were used. Robert E. Hall of the Cook County Hospital in Chicago reported in 1985 at the annual meeting of the American Academy of Orthopaedic Surgeons the results of 42 patients who were treated with modified Rush pins.[5] Eleven had isolated fracture of the radial shaft and 31 fractures of the radial and ulnar shaft. All fixations were done closed, percutaneously, and under image intensification. There were no nonunions, no malunions, no infections, no synostosis, and no implant failures, and immobilization was not used. My experience has been similar.

Basic Principles

Early treatment makes easier reduction and closed reduction and pinning simple. Semi-open techniques are used more frequently the longer it takes to perform surgery. For fractures of the proximal part of the ulna usually the pin is inserted proximally. For fractures of the ulnar and radial shaft, pins are inserted distally. The angle of insertion of the awl reamer is the key to a good reduction in three-point fixation. Distraction must be avoided for early function and healing to occur, as too long a pin is the most frequent cause of nonunion.

ULNA

The ulna is usually fractured by direct violence. It has a subcutaneous border, and there is a tendency toward displacement of the fracture toward the interosseous membrane. The ulna does not tend to shorten and overlap unless there is an associated fracture of the radius or a dislocation. The medullary canal of the ulnar is tortuous (Fig. 8–5). A longitudinal section of the bone shows it to be slightly S shaped in an anteroposterior plane. In the proximal half of the bone, in the lateral plane, there is a curvature toward the radius, whereas in the distal third of the medullary canal, it is relatively straight. The styloid process of the ulna is located posteriorly. When the forearm is in pronation, the visible and palpable bone at the wrist is the articular surface and not the styloid process.

If nonunion of this bone is to be avoided, the contour characteristics must be taken seriously into account in medullary pinning.

Fractures of the Ulna, Proximal Half

Straight ⅛-inch (3.18 mm) pins are usually used to fix fractures in the proximal half of the ulna. Insertion of the awl to the ulnar side of the oleocranon makes closed reduction and pinning much more simple. The sled runner with a slight bend is helpful, particularly if it is inserted from the radial side, which may be more convenient. With the image intensifier, the reduction is accomplished manually or by twisting the head of the pin so that the sled runner at the fracture site reduces the fracture (Fig. 8–6). The physician should be careful when determining pin length, and should not place the pin all the way into the distal part of the ulna, as distraction may occur. Fixation is usually stable, and function can be started immediately.

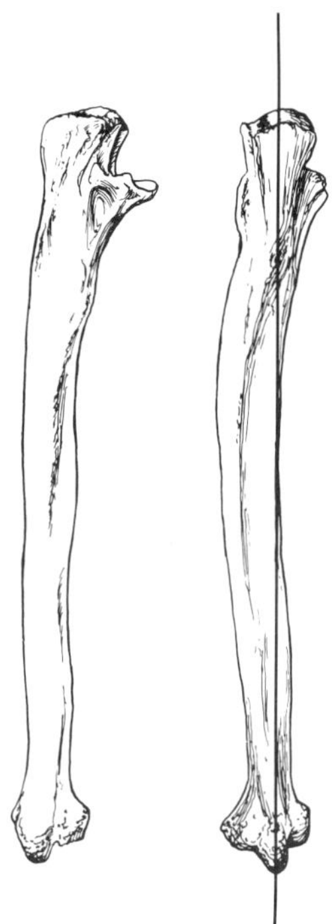

Figure 8–5. Note the radial bow of the proximal third of the ulna. The sled runner point may be needed to negotiate passage of the pin.

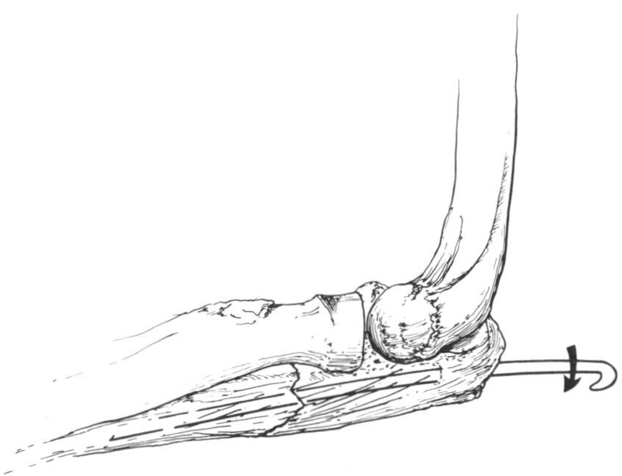

Figure 8–6. When a pin gets stuck, the point is usually trying to penetrate the cortex. Back the pin up and twist the head so that the sled runner can pass that area of the cortex.

Fractures of the Ulna, Distal Half of the Shaft

Three-point fixation is obtained by insertion of the pin in the posterior surface of the distal end of the ulna proximal to the styloid but still where cancellous bone provides entrance into the medullary canal. The direction of the awl is still 30 degrees to the proximal part of the shaft. Dynamic bending of the ⅛-inch (3.18 mm) or ³⁄₃₂-inch (2.38 mm) straight pin provides three-point fixation. It is important to bear in mind that nonunion is not infrequent in fractures of the middle third of the ulna in adults. Nonunion or patient failure to heal will usually produce pin failure. Cancellous bone grafting with exchange of the pin when a nonunion is suspected will obviate this.

When the wrist is pronated, the ulnar prominence is the articular surface of the distal radioulnar joint. With insertion of the awl in this position and the final insertion of the pin, the fracture can be reduced but the head of the pin will prevent supination (Fig. 8–7). Therefore, the awl entrance should be made with the forearm in supination when the pin is inserted from the ulnar styloid.

FRACTURES OF THE RADIAL SHAFT

For fractures of the radial shaft the site for pin insertion is usually in the snuff box near to the extensor pollicis longus (Fig. 8–8). A ⅛-inch (3.18 mm) or straight ³⁄₃₂-inch (2.38 mm) pin is used. The awl is carefully inserted so it misses the extensor tendons and the superficial branch of the radial nerve. The pin should be long enough to reach slightly proximal to the bicipital tuberosity (Fig. 8–9).

For isolated fractures of the radial shaft the semi-open technique is frequently used except for those that are done immediately because closed reduction is difficult to do. A slight bend in a distal ¼inch

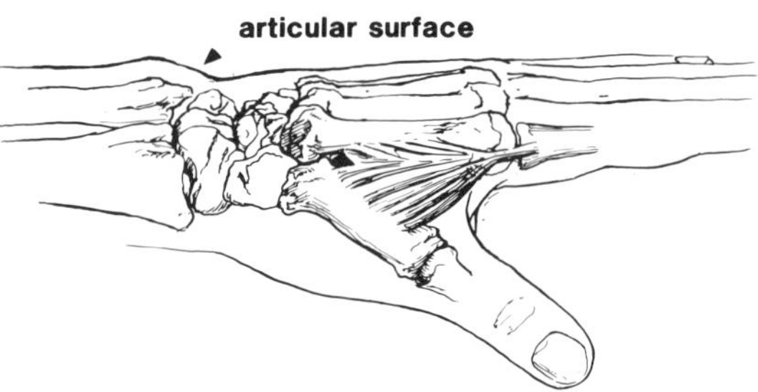

Figure 8–7. The ulnar prominence at the distal end of the forearm in the pronated position is the articular surface of the distal radioulnar joint. Do not start the awl here.

(centimeter) of a ⅛-inch (3.18 mm) pin in the same plane as the sled runner may facilitate this reduction by utilizing the pin and the sled runner to reduce the fracture. Fixation is so stable that splints are not needed and full function may be started. A Sarmiento plastic sleeve may provide additional support (Fig. 8–10).

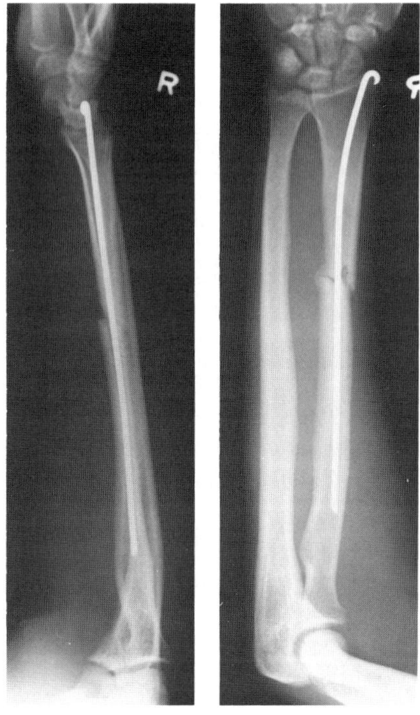

Figure 8–8. Fracture of the shaft of the radius. A 22-year-old man had closed pinning of the radius followed by stabilization with an Ace bandage and active use.

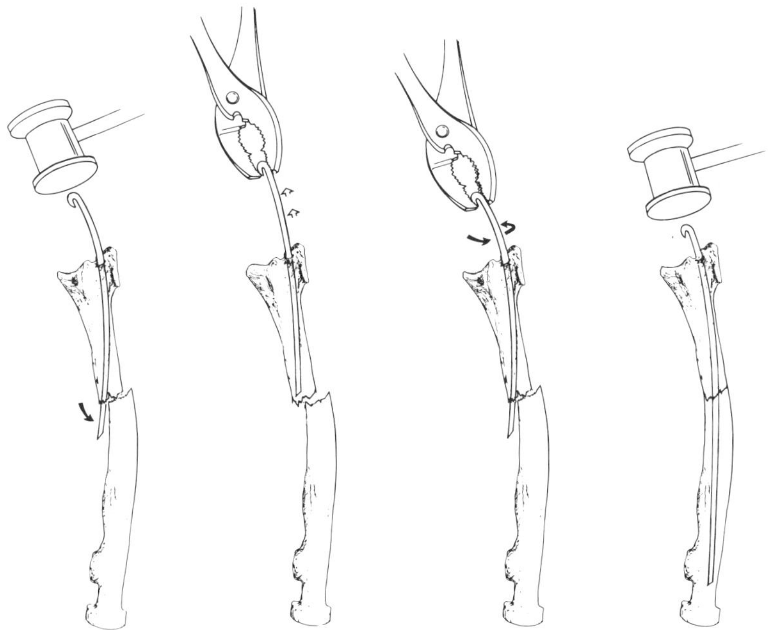

Figure 8–9.　Rotation of the sled runner by twisting the pin head may help reduce the fracture.

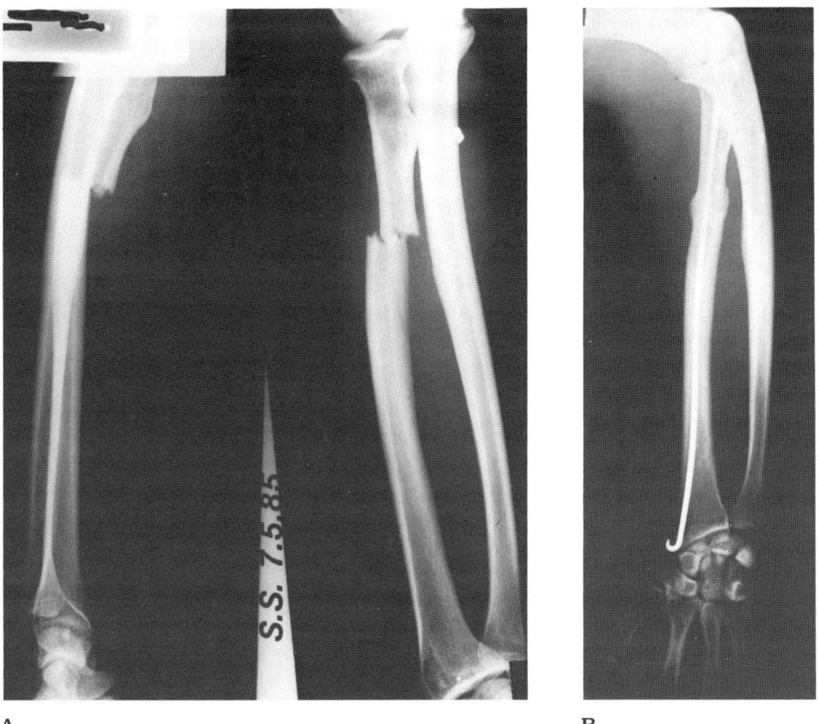

A   B

Figure 8–10.　Fracture of the proximal part of the radius. (**A**) A 37-year-old man had fracture of the humerus and proximal part of the ipsilateral radius. The radius was treated by closed pinning. (**B**) At 5 months complete healing and function were evident.

TECHNIQUE FOR FRACTURES OF BOTH BONES IN THE PROXIMAL THIRD OF THE FOREARM

Straight ⅛-inch (3.18 mm) pins are usually used with insertion from the side of the proximal aspect of the ulna and in the snuff box area of the distal end of the radius. I prefer to pin the radius first as it is usually a more difficult reduction and supination may be needed. Once the pin crosses the fracture site by approximately 1 inch, then reduction and pinning of the ulna should be attempted. One should not hesitate to use the semi-open technique.

In all fractures of bones in the forearm, one must be careful not to pin the bones in malrotation. This can cause permanent loss of rotary function of the forearm and therefore, before final seating of the pins, pronation and supination should be checked. This can be done when the pins are approximately 1 inch (2.5 cm) across the fracture site. Impaction of the pins is usually best done directly on the head of the pin itself. As the pins are impacted, the sled runner will curve from side to side as the tip slides down the medullary canal. Controlling the pin with an impactor may cause the tip of the pin to hang up in the medullary canal. If this occurs, backing up, rotating the pin with pliers, and then reinserting it is the preferred technique (Figs. 8–11, 8–12, 8–13).

TECHNIQUE FOR FRACTURES OF BOTH BONES IN THE DISTAL THIRD OF THE FOREARM

Insertion of straight ⅛-inch (3.18 mm) pins through the styloid into the radius

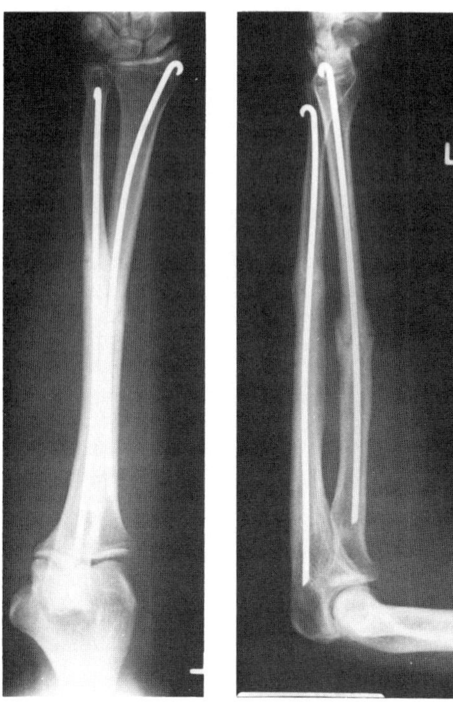
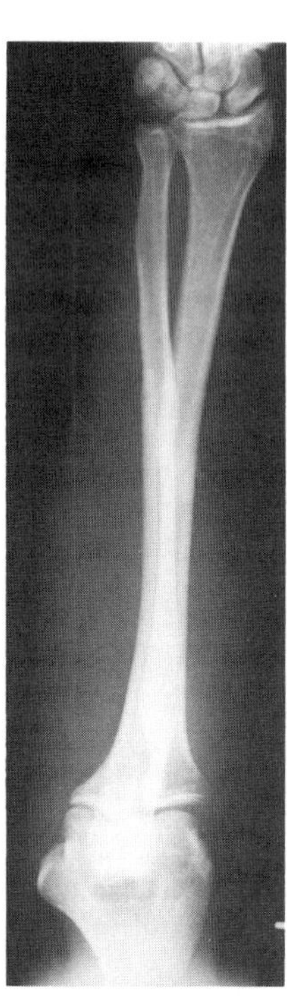
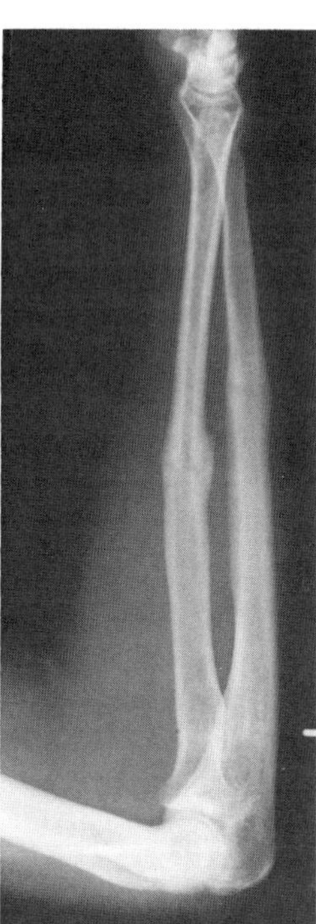

A   B

Figure 8–11. Fracture disease. Anterior-posterior and lateral radiographs show: **(A)** Both fractures in the forearm are healed, and the arm has full range of motion. **(B)** There is no sign of fracture disease after pin removal.

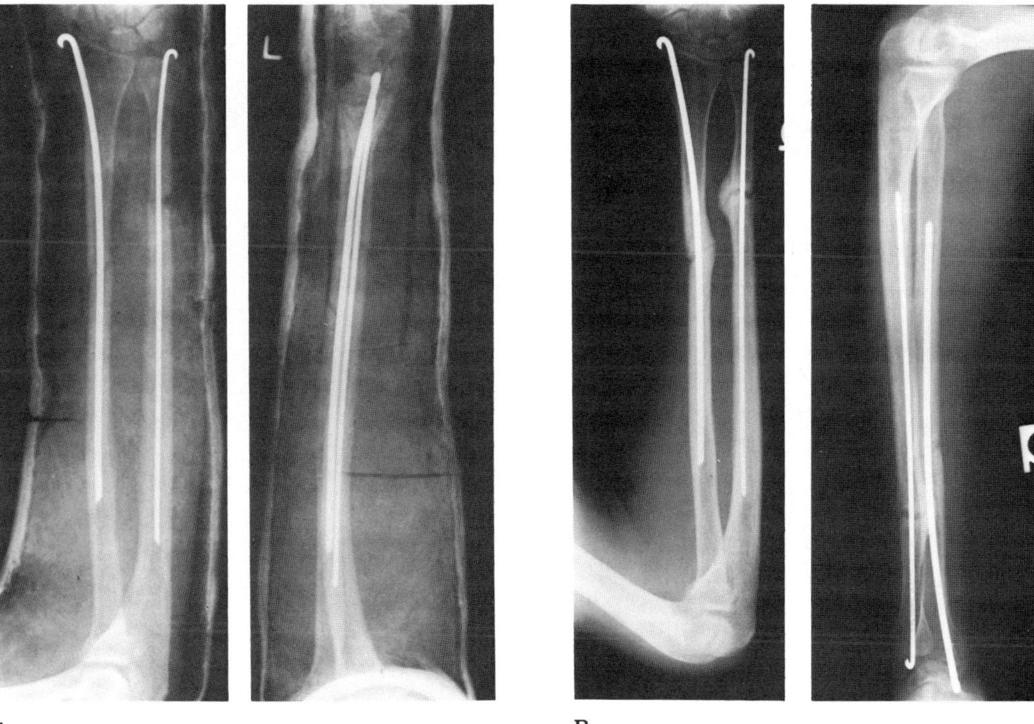

A   B

Figure 8–12.   Open fracture in the forearm (**A**) A 20-year-old man had Gustilo Grade II open fractures of the radius and ulna. The fractures were debrided and pinned with ⅛-inch (3.18 mm) and ³⁄₃₂-inch (2.38 mm) pins in July 1972. (**B**) Fractures healed and the arm had almost full function in June 1973.

and from the styloid area of the ulna has been previously mentioned. Both pins should be long enough to go into the proximal third of the radius and ulna but not into the articular surface. The fracture of the radius is first reduced, and the pin is driven across the fracture into the proximal fragment for about an inch. The ulnar fracture is then reduced, and the ulnar pin is driven across the fragments into the proximal fragment for about an inch. Pronation and supination are performed with the arm under the image intensifier, and the pins are competely inserted within ½ inch (12.72 mm) of the skin and then finally inserted with an impactor. Stability is usually good, and a Sarmiento sleeve may be used if there is a question, but most frequently use of an elastic bandage and early function is the treatment of choice. Oblique fractures of

the distal part of the radius make three-point fixation difficult and it is not accomplished well unless the end of the pin is sharply stress relieved. Please refer to Chapter 4 for the formula in this situation. The only situation is to stress relieve the proximal pin or add a cerclage wire.

TECHNICAL CONSIDERATIONS

An oblique fracture in the distal fragment of a portion of the radius makes three-point fixation difficult and is not accomplished unless the pin in the short fragment is sharply stress relieved.

A bulbous radial styloid makes insertion of the pin difficult. The pin site must be closer to Lister's tubercle.

In fractures of the distal part of the ulnar shaft, it is best to insert the pin

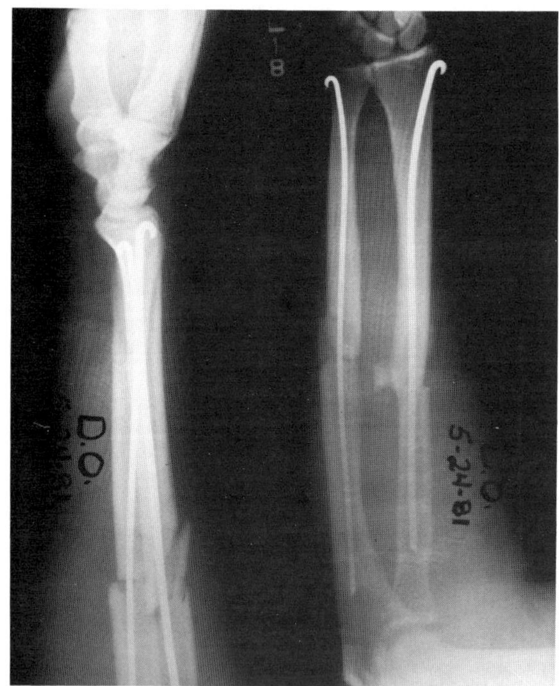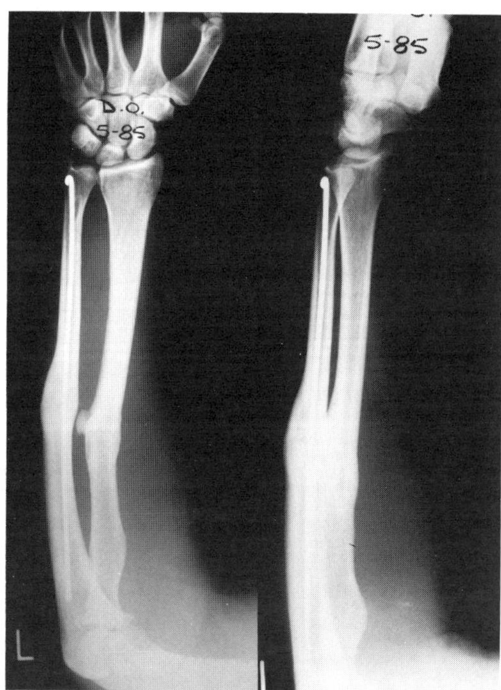

A   B

Figure 8–13. Fracture of both shafts. (**A**) A male racetrack driver had open tibial and fibular fractures and comminuted fractures of the forearm midshafts. Semi-open technique was performed on the radius and ulna and a fiberglass cast was worn. The driver returned to racing in 4 months. (**B**) These radiographs were made 4 years later.

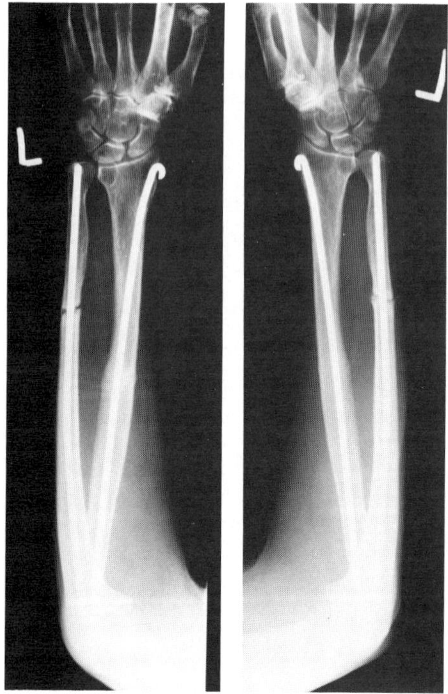

A   B

Figure 8–14. Effects of distraction with long ulnar pin. (**A**) An 82-year-old man had a pin inserted from olecranon that was too long in July 1982. (**B**) This is the same forearm in March 1983. The radius healed and remodeled. The ulna slowly healed (continued).

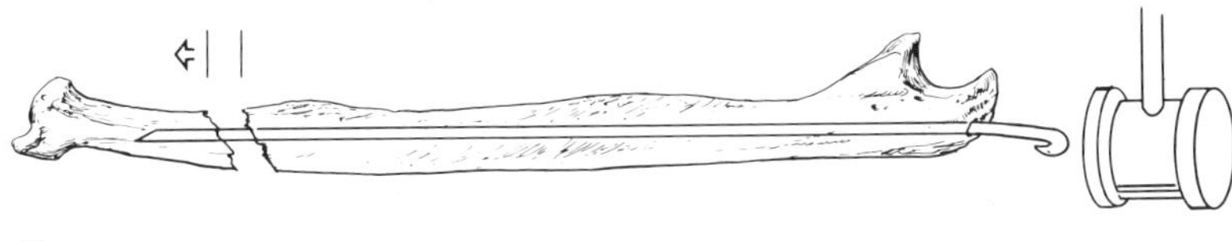

C

Figure 8–14 (cont.).   (C) was inserted from the olecranon to treat a fracture of the distal part of the ulna. This frequently distracts the fracture.

from the styloid or distal end of the ulna to prevent distraction of the fracture (Fig. 8–14).

Incomplete reduction of one bone of the forearm can produce distraction of the fellow bone.

REFERENCES

1. Rush, L.D., Rush, H.L. A reconstruction operation for a comminuted fracture of the upper third of the ulna. Am. Jnl. Surg:38:332–333, 1937.
2. Sage, F.: Medullary fixation of forearm fractures. J. Bone Joint Surg. 41A:1489–1516, 1959.
3. Caden, J.G.: Internal fixation of fractures of the forearm. J. Bone Joint Surg. 43A:1115–1121, 1961.
4. Aho, A.J., Nieminen, S.J., Salo, U., Luoma, R.: Antebrachium fractures: Rush pin fixation today in the light of late results. J. Trauma 24(7):604–610, 1984.
5. Hall, R.E.: Presented at the annual meeting of the American Academy of Orthopaedic Surgeons, Las Vegas, Nevada Jan 27, 1985.

SUGGESTED READINGS

Ono, M., Bechtold, J.E., Merkow, R.L., et al.: Rotational stability of diaphyseal fractures of the radius and ulna fixed with compression plates, Rush pins, and/or fracture bracing. Orthop. Trans. 11(2):295–296, 1987.
Rush, L.V.: Atlas of Rush Pin Technics. Meridian, Mississippi, The Berivon Company, 1955.

CHAPTER 9

Colles' and Distal Radial Fractures

Indications:
  Bilateral Colles' Fractures
  Colles' Fractures with Carpal Tunnel Syndrome
  Comminuted Colles' Fractures
  Colles' Fractures with Skin Burns, Abrasions or Loss of Skin
Reduction
Technique
Reverse Colles' or Smith's Fracture
Barton's Fracture
Colles' Fracture with Ulna Fracture at the Same Level
Fractures with Carpal Tunnel Syndrome
Pitfalls

At the 1968 meeting of the American Fracture Association, I presented a series of 74 Colles' fractures in 73 patients, all treated by closed reduction and internal fixation with ³⁄₃₂-inch (2.38 mm) Rush pins. The average age of the patients was 79 years the patients were primarily female, and the fractures were on the left side. Three fractures were open. There were no infections, and no nonunions. Six pins were left too long. One pin was inserted into a fracture and migrated into the medullary canal. There were two injuries to the superficial branch of the radial nerve on removal of the pin. Two patients had associated injuries to the median nerve. One patient had a fracture of the scaphoid.

Various methods of anesthesia that were tried included local injection, axillary nerve block, supraclavicular nerve block, Bier block, general anesthetic, and general anesthetic with injection of local anesthetic at the fracture site. The best anesthesia for outpatient treatment is axillary nerve block because of its long-lasting effect. The best in a teaching situation is general anesthesia with injection of 2% lidocaine at the fracture site. This allows for comfort and early function after general anesthesia and allows the procedure to be done on an outpatient basis. The best indications for the use of Rush pin fixation in Colles' fractures are:

1. Bilateral Colles' fractures
2. Colles' fracture with median nerve injury
3. Comminuted Colles' fractures
4. Colles' fracture with severe skin abrasions, burns, or skin loss

THE TECHNIQUE OF TREATMENT

1. The patient is given the usual skin preparation, usually alcohol and Betadine spray (povidone-iodine) that is allowed to dry.
2. Injection of the fracture site with 10 ml of 2% lidocaine is done. in addition to adequate anesthesia.
3. the method of reduction of fracture that I prefer, since it is easy, is a triangulation method using my elbow against the patient's arm and then with direct pressure and with the opposite hand, the triangle is changed to put rather marked traction on the distal end of the Colles' fracture. This easily gives length and the dorsal angulation can be reduced with direct pressure. Palpation will usually tell if a fracture is reduced. Obviously, all methods of traction and manipulation rely on the radial carpal ligaments, both volar and dorsal, to reduce the fracture. This is one of the reasons why comminuted fractures still can be pinned as the bony pieces are held by their connecting radial carpal ligaments.

4. By holding the fracture reduced with one hand, the physician can palpate the snuff box area, and a 3-mm incision is made through the distal skin of the radius over the radial scaphoid articulation.
5. A short ³⁄₃₂-inch (2.38 mm) awl is placed vertically to the skin to palpate the joint between the scaphoid and the radius (Figs. 9–1, 9–2). Then the tip is placed on the dorsal surface of the radius in this area, and a hole is made with the awl. The awl is inserted and then gradually changed to a 30 degree angle to the longitudinal axis. One must understand that the center of the radioscaphoid joint in the lunate is not in the center of the longitudinal axis of the radius but is slightly more volar so that insertion of the pin must be dorsal to the mid-axis of the radioscaphoid and lunate joint. The juxta-articular bone is always the most dense and is covered with the radiocarpal ligament. This is why the area should be used for insertion of the awl and the pin. The physician should avoid putting the awl into the radial styloid as it is too volar, and the

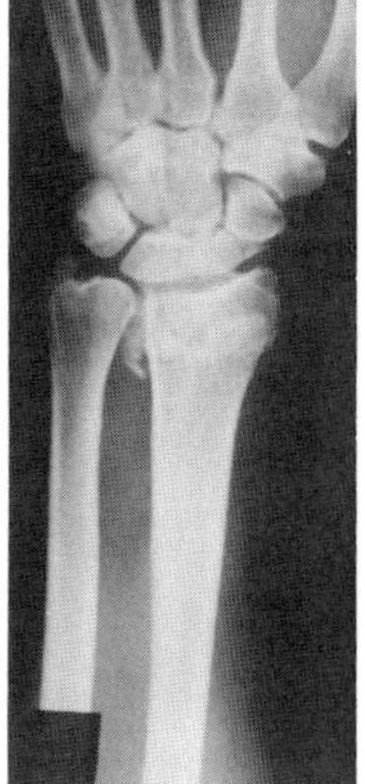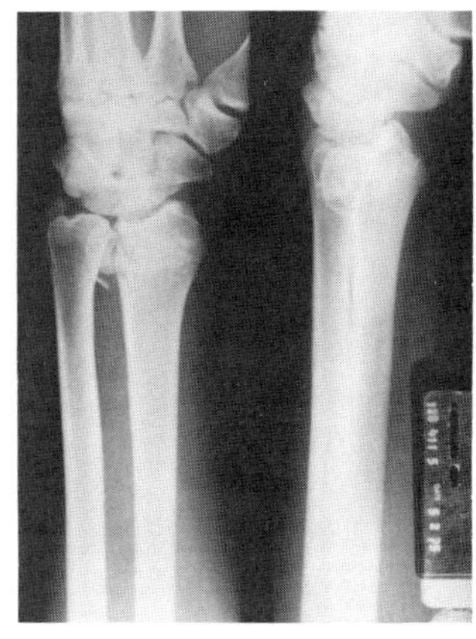

A

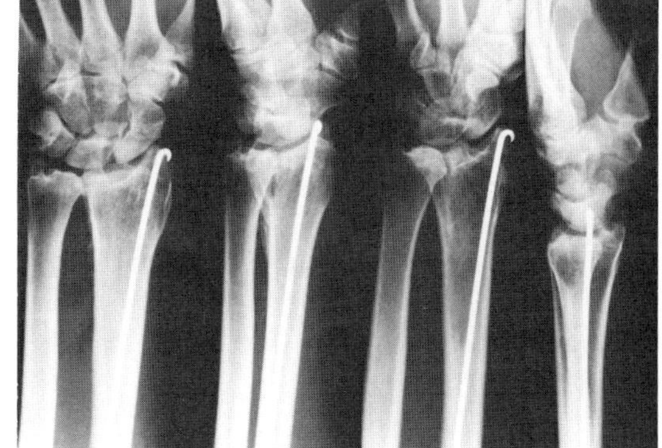

B

Figure 9–1. Colles' fracture. **(A)** A 56-year-old man had a comminuted Colles' fracture and a fracture of the middle third of the waist scaphoid. A closed reduction with pinning was done and a thumb spica was applied for 6 weeks. **(B)** The navicular fracture healed and early active motion was initiated.

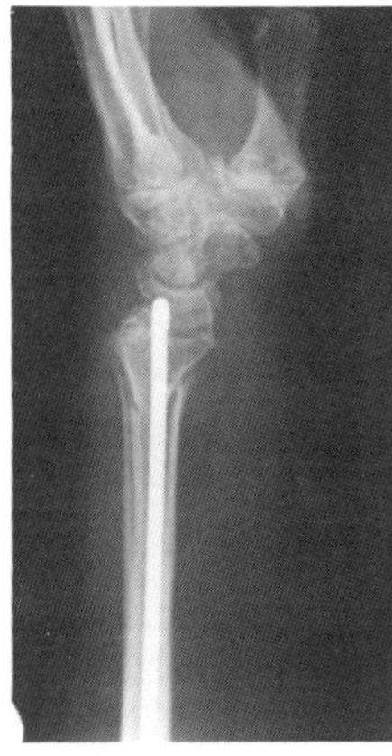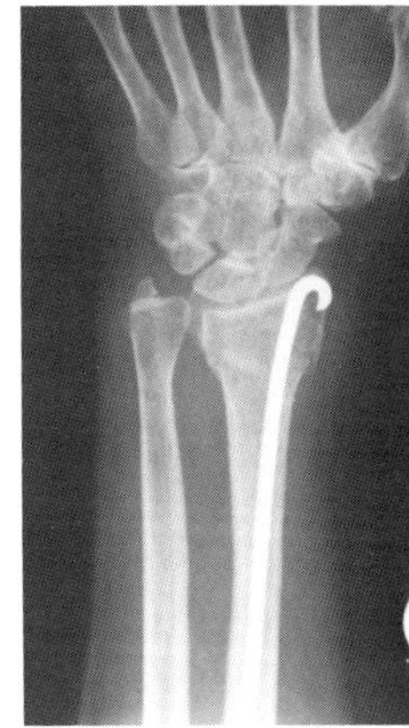

Figure 9–2. A 78-year-old woman who was visiting Meridian, Mississippi, in 1983 suffered a displaced Colles' fracture and was treated by Dr. Leslie V. Rush, Sr., and returned to the Indianapolis area. The sutures were removed and active use was continued; no cast was applied.

pin will produce reangulation of the fracture.

6. The usual pin length is P (13.97 cm), Q (15.24 cm), R (16.51 cm) in the ³⁄₃₂-inch (2.38 mm) Rush pin. Every set should have at least a 2½- to 3-inch-long (7.62 cm) ³⁄₃₂-inch (2.38 mm) pin for the narrow medullary canal usually found in young females. One-eighth-inch (3.18 mm) pins are too resilient, and I find it difficult to stress relieve them, so I use them infrequently.

7. The pin is exchanged with the awl by sliding down the awl slot into the radius, and then it is pushed in about an inch.

8. At this time, manual reduction is again palpated, and if satisfactory, the pin is pushed into the proximal part of the medullary canal. In the older patient, the pin can be pushed a good share of the way, and one can feel the sled runner grate down the medullary canal. The grating sensation saves the need for a radiograph, as it always means that the pin is intramedullary.

9. When the pin is within 3 inches of final seating, the fracture starts to become stable. The sound of impaction with the mallet changes, and the pin is further inserted until it almost disappears in the incision.

10. Radiographs are taken in anteroposterior and lateral planes for confirmation.

11. The pin is then impacted so the hook is barely palpable at the distal end of the radius and the skin is closed with a single suture.

12. Simple fractures are then treated with an adhesive bandage and an elastic bandage. For comminuted fractures a dorsal plaster splint is usually applied and held in place with an elastic bandage.

13. Postoperative course is important as early function is mandatory, especially finger motion at the proximal interphalangeal joints. Wrist motion usually takes a few weeks before it is done with ease, and one should not worry about this.

14. Fracture healing takes the usual 6 to 8 weeks and strengthening is possible by exercises, squeezing a ball, or preferably Play-Doh, a children's putty.

SMITH OR REVERSE COLLES' FRACTURE

The technique for Smith fracture fixation is similar to that for Colles' fracture except that the pin is inserted on the volar surface between the insertion of the brachioradialis, the abductor pollicis longus, and the radial artery. Because of the swelling associated with the fracture and the location of the radial artery, a ¾-inch (2.0 cm) incision is made to locate the interval between the artery and the tendon, and the awl is inserted in a similar manner but on the volar aspect. Postoperative management is the same as for the Colles' fracture.

BARTON'S FRACTURE

The Barton's fracture is associated with a dislocation of the carpus and a rather small radial articular lip, and this can be a vexing problem because of the tendency for redislocation. I have found the best approach to be visualization of the fracture site with minimal dissection and then insertion of a (2.38 mm) awl into the fracture site and ultimate insertion of a P, Q, or R length 3⁄32-inch (2.38 mm) pin, which is then left protruding across the dorsal aspect of the carpus by approximately ½ inch (12.72 mm). This will hold the reduction for a few weeks until removal of the pin is possible. Removal of the pin can be done under local anesthesia, with such a long portion of pin palpable. The reverse or volar type of Barton's fracture is handled similarly but the pin always needs to be removed, and it is much more of a surgical undertaking.

COLLES' FRACTURE WITH THE ULNA FRACTURED AT THE SAME LEVEL

Colles' fracture with the ulna fractured at the same level can be a problem, for the resilient pin in the radius needs a balancing ulnar buttress. In the treatment of this fracture, after manual reduction, the ulna should be treated first and then the Colles' fracture treated in the usual manner. It is important that after reduction, the wrist be held in supination and the ulnar awl inserted near or at the styloid process. Insertion of the awl with the wrist pronated will put the pin in the articular surface of the distal radioulnar joint, and while it can hold the fracture satisfactorily, it will prevent supination until the pin is removed. After the pin is inserteed with the fracture in its reduced position and the wrist in supination, the

wrist can be held as one would treat a normal Colles' fracture and the procedure completed.

FRACTURES WITH CARPAL TUNNEL SYNDROME

Although the series is small, the acute median nerve syndrome can be greatly averted by injecting the carpal tunnel with a steroid after reduction and pinning of the fracture. A cast should be avoided.

PITFALLS

Insertion of the pin must not be in the fracture site. The juxta-articular bone with ligamentous attachments is still the best point of insertion. The ulna must be a buttress, for the resilient pin placed in the distal part of the radius will push against the ulna, and it will angulate. The awl reamer angle must be 30 degrees.

TRAVERSING THE SHORT FRAGMENT

To transfix any short fragment, the point chosen for insertion must be accurate. The pin must traverse the short fragment in line closely approaching the long axis of the medullary canal. Otherwise, deflection of the pin in the medullary canal will force the fragment into malposition or angulation.

In Colles' fracture, the wrong angle of insertion in the short fragment can produce anterior angulation, posterior angulation, or ulnar deviation of the fragment. In other regions, similar deformity can be produced. If the pin is not opposed by intrinsic forces, the pin must be opposed by the force of a second pin (Fig. 9–3).

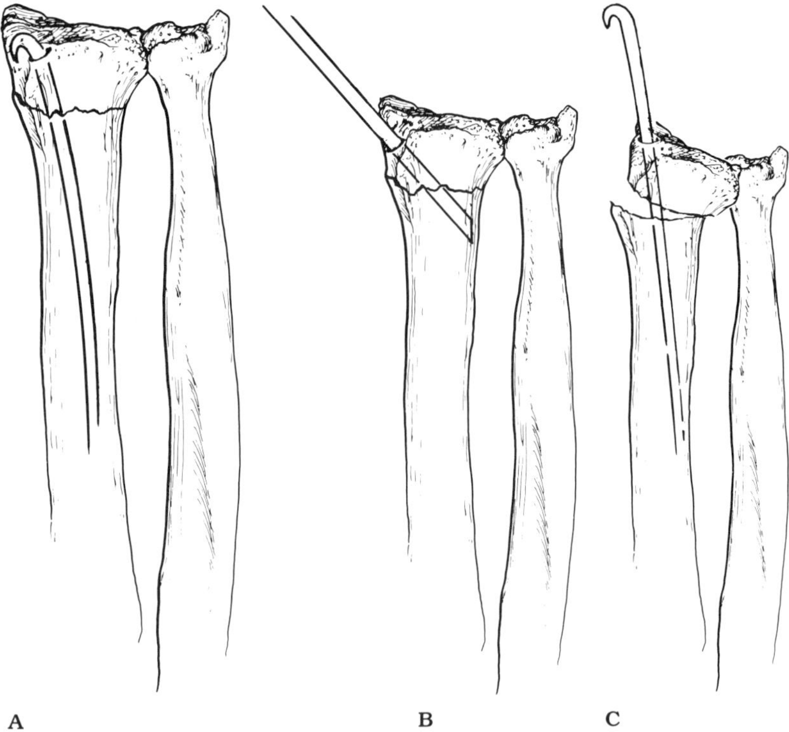

Figure 9–3.   Transversing the short fragment. (**A**) Correct: Pin has been properly applied in an axis approximating that of the medullary cavity. (**B**) Wrong: Point of insertion will produce deformity. (**C**) Wrong: Angle of insertion will produce ulnar deviation of fragment.

SUGGESTED READINGS

Lucas, G.L., Sachtjen, K.M.: An analysis of hand function in patients with Colles' fractures treated by Rush pins. Clin. Orthop. 155:172–179, 1981.

Rush, L.V.: Atlas of Rush Pin Technics. Meridian, Mississippi, The Berivon Company, 1956.

Rush, L.V.: Closed medullary pinning of Colles' fractures. Clin. Orthop. 3:152–162, 1954.

Thornton, L., Warner, P.: The management of Colles' fractures with the Rush medullary nail. South. Med. J. 48:854–857, 1955.

Fractures About the Ankle

The key to diagnosing fractures of the ankle relates to the forces of the talus that produce the final fracture.

Classification of ankle fractures is necessary for communication between physicians and for comparison of results. There are three classification systems: The Ashhurst and Bromer classification,[1] 1922, primarily involves external rotation forces, abduction forces, adduction forces, and compression forces. The Lauge-Hansen classification,[2] 1949–1954, uses supination-eversion (external rotation forces), pronation-eversion (external rotation), supination-adduction forces, pronation-abduction forces, and pronation-dorsiflexion forces.

The Danis-Weber classification[3] is based on the appearance and the location of the fibular fracture. It does not permit categorization according to severity, however. The Danis-Weber Type A corresponds to the supination-adduction. Type B corresponds to the supination-external rotation and the pronation-abduction mechanism. The Danis-Weber Type C, a fracture above the syndesmosis and rupture of the tibiofibular ligament, corresponds to pronation-external rotation.

Ligamentous injury plays a great role in stability and location of the fracture is the key as to what ligaments are torn. In the Danis-Weber Type C fracture, complete tibiotalar ligamentous tears including the interosseous membrane are present. The Danis-Weber Type B fracture shows partial tibiofibular ligamentous disruption.

Nothing replaces clinical evaluation under adequate anesthesia to determine ankle stability. Palpation over a painful deltoid ligament as well as the fibular ligaments and normal appearance on radiographs must lead to the conclusion of ligamentous injury. As mentioned by Yablon and others,[4] the talus follows the fibular fracture and reduction is most important.

OSTEOLOGY

The fibular malleolus has a pyramidal shape, somewhat flattened from side to side. The medial surface is triangular and covered with articular surface. The lateral surface is subcutaneous. The anterior surface is rough and covered with ligaments, and the posterior surface is notched with the malleolus sulcus holding the peroneal tendons. The proximal end of the medullary canal narrows rapidly above the level of the syndesmosis, and passage of an intramedullary pin is dependent on proper insertion of the awl reamer and getting the sled runner to bounce off the opposite cortex before proceeding into the intramedullary canal.

Fortunately, in the Danis-Weber Type B fracture, or supination-external rotation fracture, the spiral fibula is usually in the plane from anterior inferior to posterior superior so that using the formula for victory produces solid stabilization when a Rush pin is properly placed. The victory formula (Chapter 4) is: When a pin is inserted in the short fragment to transfix an oblique fracture near the end of the extremity of the bone, the pin should be directed so that the axis of the shaft of the pin tends to parallel the axis of the fracture line.

The fibular malleolus is fixed with a straight ⅛-inch (3.18 mm) pin (Fig. 10–1). It is inserted in the malleolus at its anterolateral surface behind the syndesmotic ligaments, at the subcutaneous border for most fractures with an oblique fracture line. The awl reamer is aimed by a scooping action pointing 20 to 30 degrees to the fibular axis, with care not to insert it too deeply (Fig. 10–2A). The straight ⅛inch (3.18 mm) pin with its sled runner will deflect off the medial cortex and up the medullary canal (Fig. 10–2B). If the awl reamer is not exactly correct, a slight bend in the same plane as the sled runner using a bending iron will

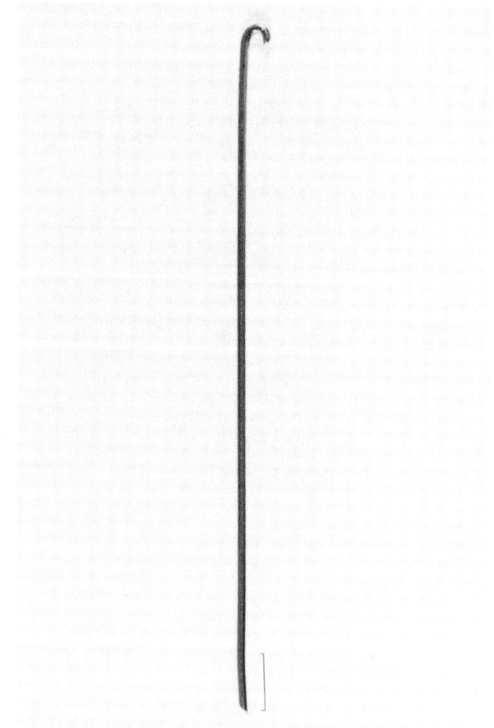

Figure 10–1. The ⅛-inch (3.18 mm) or ³⁄₃₂-inch (2.38 mm) Rush pin is more easily passed across the fracture if the distal ½-inch (12.72 mm) has a slight angular bend to it.

allow passage into the proximal part of the fibula (Fig. 10–1).

The resilient pin, in its dynamic position in soft bone, will need to be stress relieved using the bending iron to keep the head from migrating into the intermedullary canal (Figs. 10–3, 10–4).

DANIS-WEBER TYPE C FRACTURES WITH DIASTASIS

With the fracture of the fibula above the syndesmosis, a straight ⅛-inch (3.18 mm) fibular pin is placed across the syndesmosis into the tibia from the lateral side and the pin stress relieved using the bending iron. The pin going across the syndesmosis is then supplemented

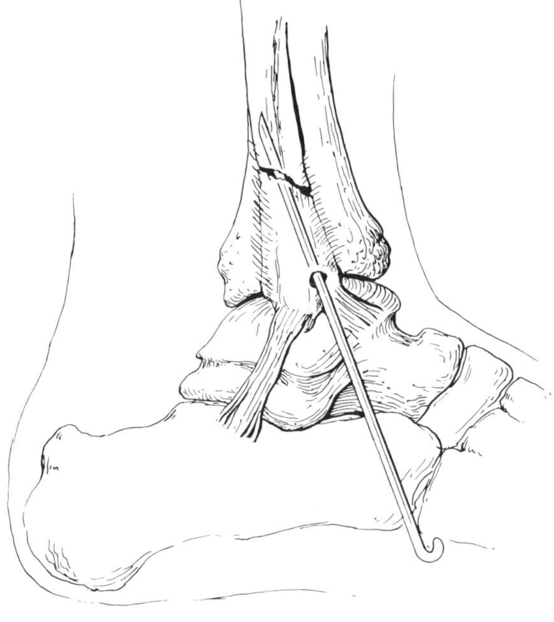

A

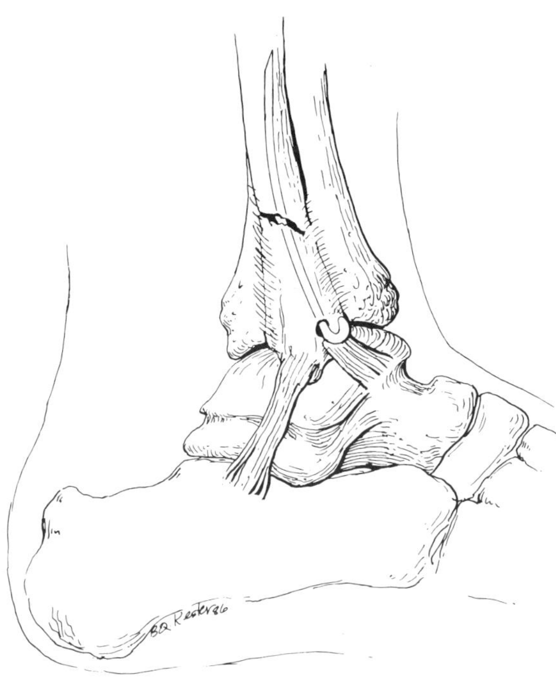

B

Figure 10–2. **(A)** The straight pin with the tip end slightly bent is inserted through an awl hole in the anterolateral surface of the fibular malleolus across the fracture site. **(B)** The pin develops a slight bend as it becomes dynamically inserted.

with an additional pin in the fibula, usually more distally located than this and up the medullary canal as previously described (Fig. 10–5). The blood supply and soft-tissue envelope is not usually disturbed and early function with a sugar tong splint is the rule.

Healing is evident by the formation of callus at the fracture site.

Removal of the fibular pin is relatively simple, and active use of a load-sharing device allows minimal restrictions after removal of the metal.

COMMINUTED FRACTURES

These fractures can be treated by minimal dissection and use of cerclage wire for retubulation and a longer pin (Fig. 10–6). Fixation utilizes the interosseous membrane and stabilization in the medullary canal to maintain length. Leach,[5] in 1964, demonstrated that fibular fixation is able to hold tibial fractures to length (Fig. 10–7).

SUPRAMALLEOLAR OR TIBIAL PILON FRACTURES

Supramalleolar fractures are usually associated with high-velocity accidents (Figs. 10–8, 10–9). Generally the fibula is fractured at or above the tibial plafond. It is a serious injury, with intra-articular fractures and soft-tissue disruption being quite common. The fractures are similar to all articular fractures near joints, particularly the Colles' fracture, the supracondylar femoral fracture, and fracture of the tibial plateau, in that the soft-tissue ligamentous support helps reduce the articular surfaces and is important in preserving for early function.

Leach[5] described fixation of the fibula

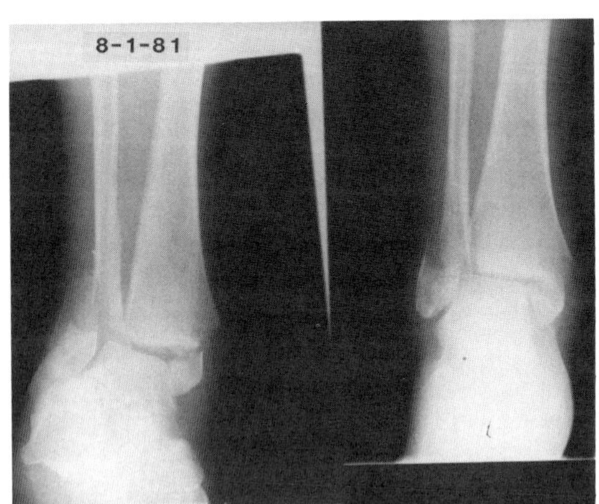
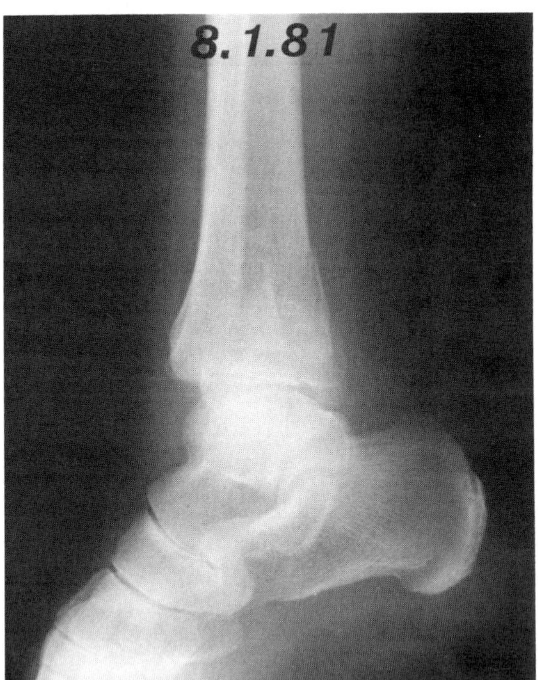

A

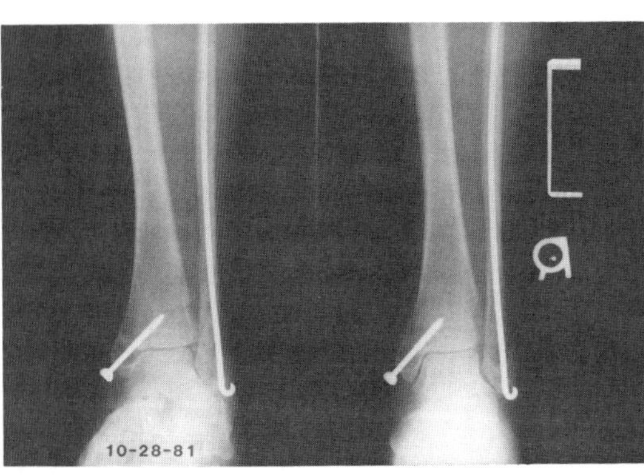
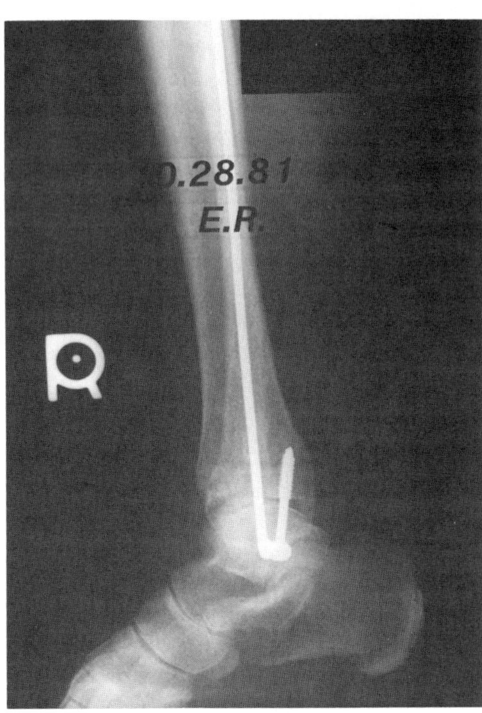

B

Figure 10–3.   (A) A 55-year-old woman suffered a displaced trimalleolar fracture at the ankle on August 1, 1981. She was taken to surgery where the fibular fracture was treated with a Rush pin and an AO malleolar screw for the medial malleolus. (B) Follow-up radiographs made on October 28, 1981, show the fracture healed, without evidence of fracture disease and with a normal range of motion.

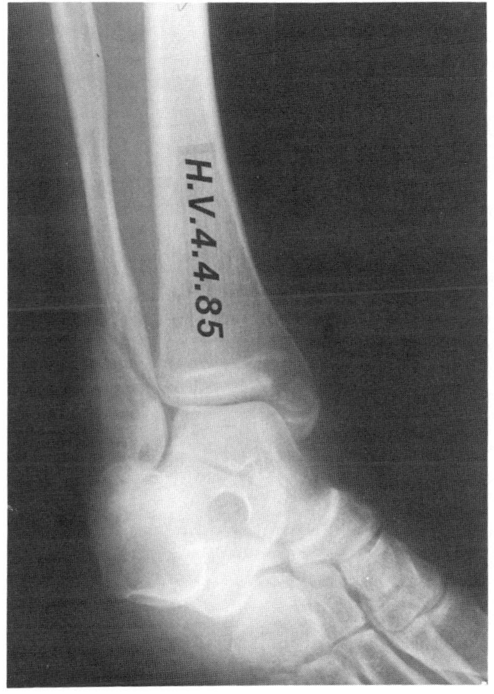

A

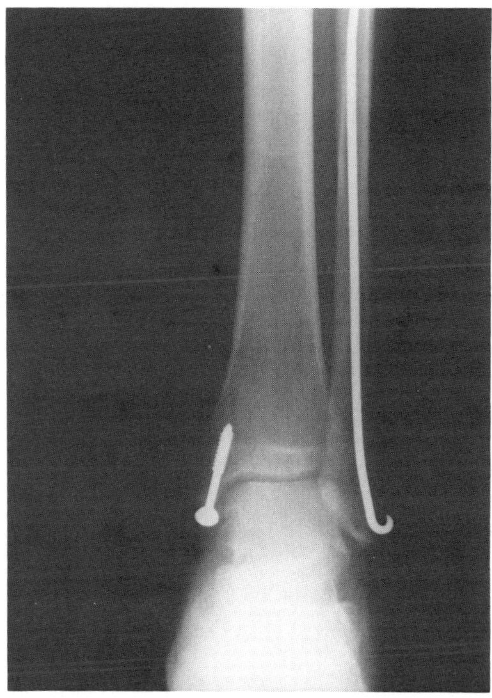

B

Figure 10–4. (A) A 68-year-old man had a displaced bimalleolar fracture at the ankle. (B) Treatment was with pin and screw fixation and early active ankle motion. Prompt healing occurred. Note the slight curve in the tip end of the pin.

with the Rush pin, but this fracture can be managed with a percutaneous pin with or without cerclage wires.

Occasionally two ⅛-inch (3.18 mm) pins in the distal end of the tibia used in the manner as for supracondylar femoral fractures are helpful in controlling fixation (Fig. 10–11A). The area of insertion is most important, and first straight ⅛-inch (3.18 mm) pins should be inserted after the awl reamer has been placed in the anterior tubercle of Tillaux-Chaput, and by manipulating the ankle into a varus deformity, the pin is impacted so that it goes into the proximal part of the medullary canal (Fig. 10–11B). After this, a second ⅛-inch (3.18 mm) tibial pin is inserted at the level proximal to the medial malleolus using the awl reamer; this will allow the pin to become intramedullary without too much difficulty. The pins are then impacted alternately. The fibula is then pinned as mentioned in a previously described fashion.

John Reynolds, M.D., provided me with this excellent result of percutaneous pinning in a Gustilo Type III open fracture with supplemental external pin fixation and a cast to provide the proper angle of the tibial plafond (Fig. 10–12).

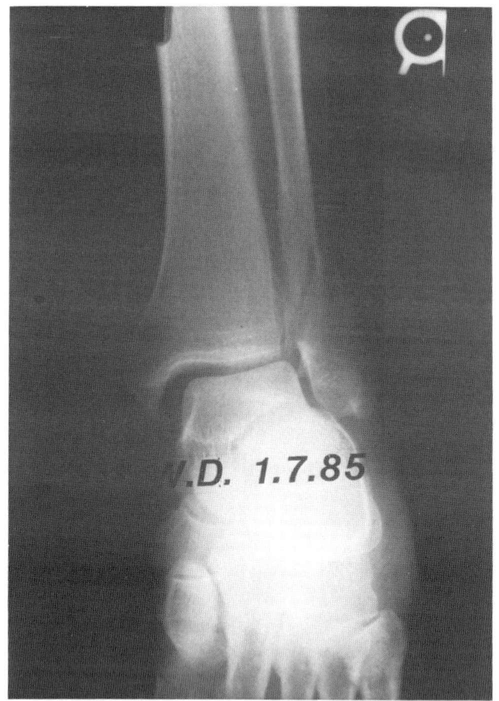

Figure 10–5. (**A**) A patient had a spiral fracture of the fibula and widening of the ankle mortise on January 7, 1985. Closed reduction was attempted, but failed. (**B**) In 1 week, the fracture was treated surgically with dynamic pin fixation in the fibula, which closed the ankle mortise. Prompt healing and full range of motion were achieved by April 8, 1985.

A

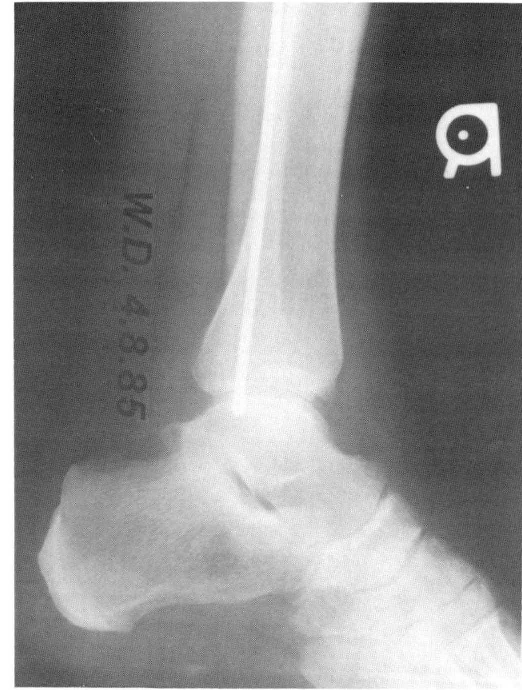

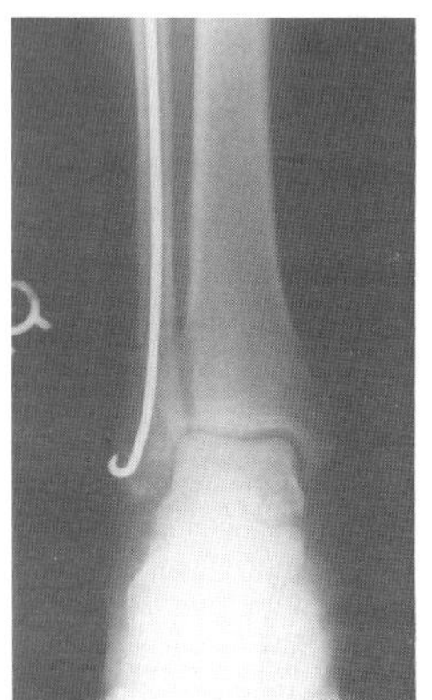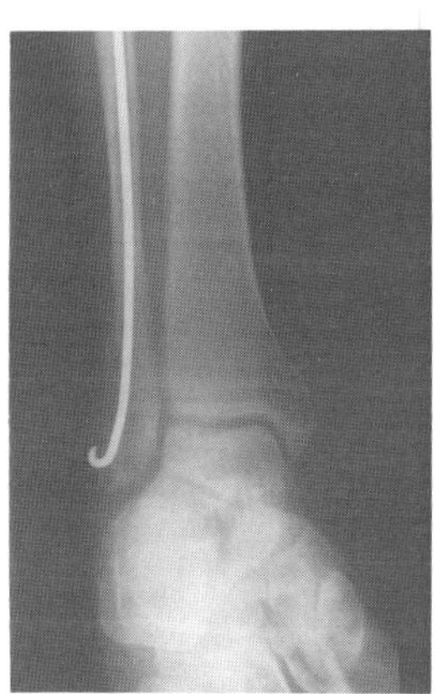

B

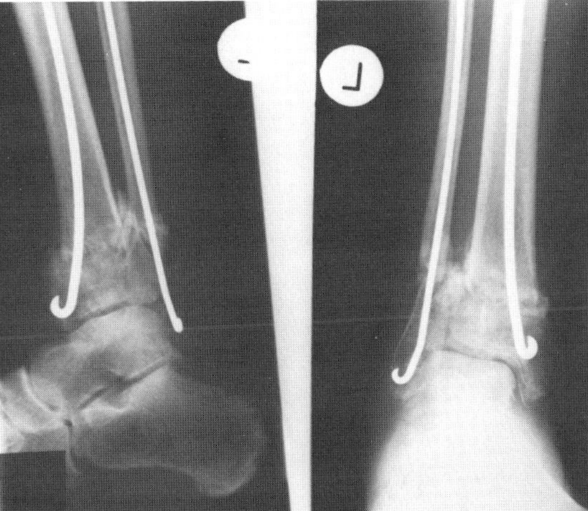

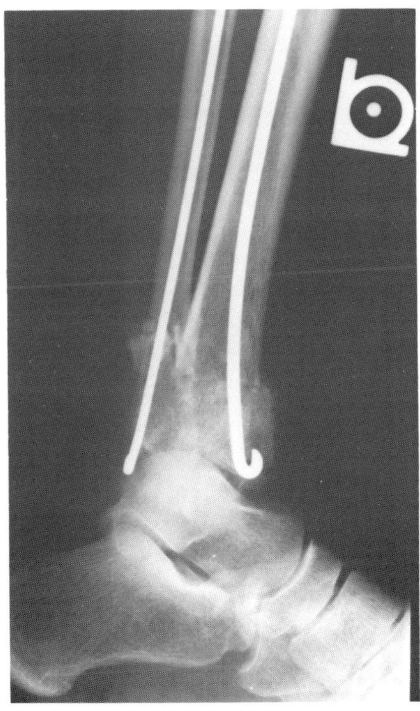

Figure 10–6. Comminuted fracture. 3 radiographic views A 65-year-old woman had a comminuted supramalleolar fracture at the left ankle treated by closed pinning with a ³⁄₃₂-inch (2.38 mm) fibula rpin and a ⅛-inch (3.18 mm) pin to the medial distal aspect of the tibia. Healing was slow, but progressive, in 10 weeks.

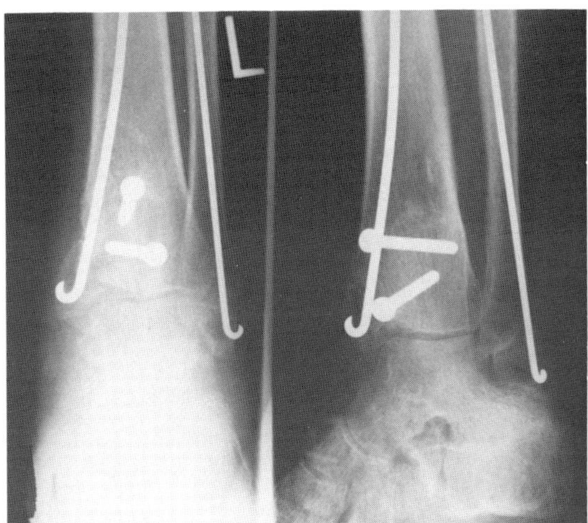

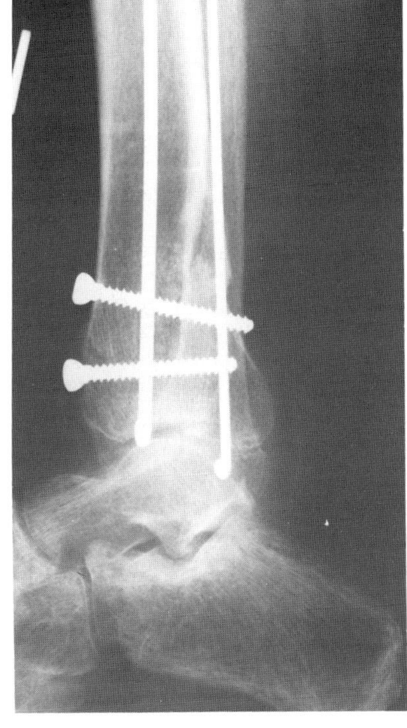

Figure 10–7. A 62-year-old man had a comminuted displaced trimalleolar fracture at the ankle treated with a ³⁄₃₂-inch (2.38 mm) fibular pin and two AO 4.5 mm screws placed anteriorly for the posterior malleolus and ⅛-inch (3.18 mm) dynamic pin to maintain length of the medial side. The patient wore a cast for 7 weeks and then was allowed partial weight-bearing. 3 radiographic views demonstrate fixation

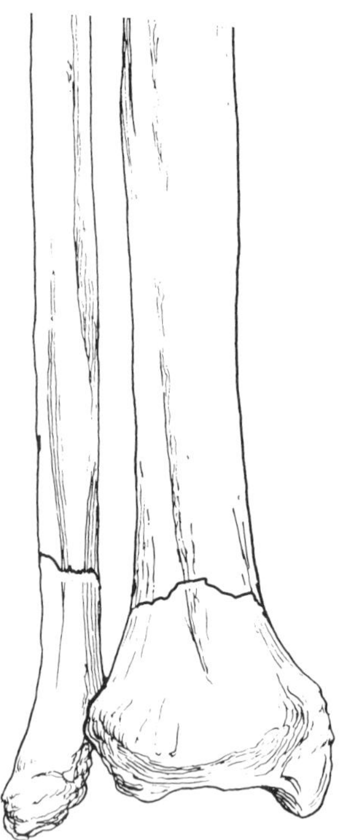

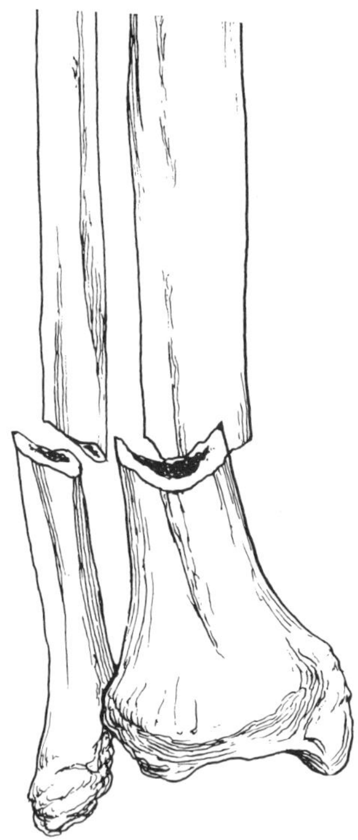

Figure 10–8. Undisplaced supramalleolar fractures may be stable.

Figure 10–9. Displaced supramalleolar fractures are unstable, frequently with contused soft tissue.

Figure 10–10. A supramalleolar fracture, similar to that in Figure 10–6 but without the fibular fracture, is more difficult to manage but still possible by using dynamic pin fixation.

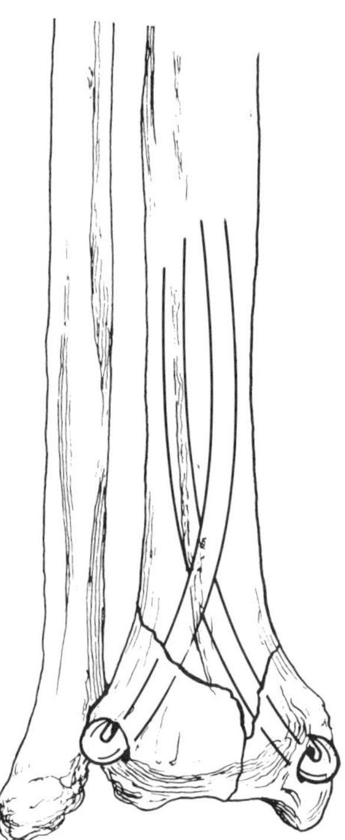

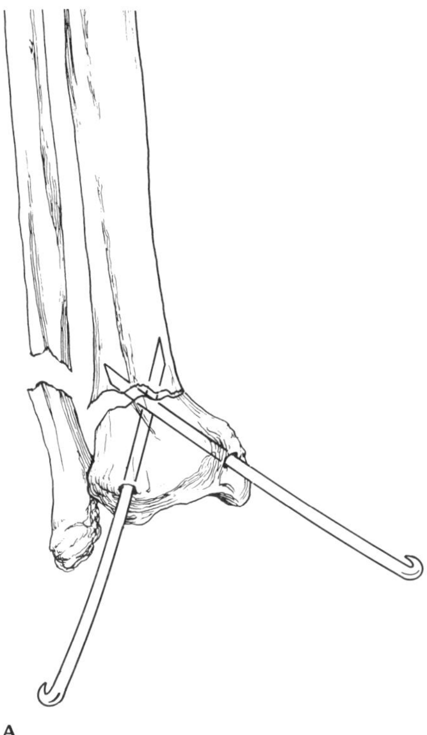

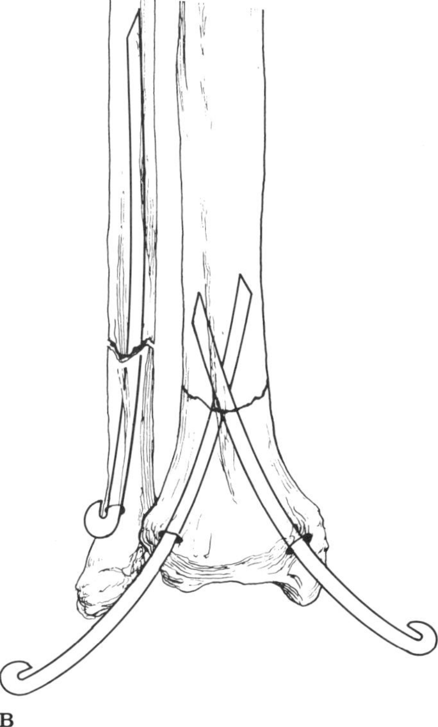

Figure 10–11. Supramalleolar fractures are similar to supracondylar fractures. (**A**) The awl is started in the lateral supramalleolar area at an angle as close to the foot as possible. The pin can pass into the tibia by bending the fracture into varus position to get the pin across, then reducing the fracture and pinning from the medial side. (**B**) The straight pins when further impacted develop a dynamic curve and firm fixation. The fibula can be pinned then.

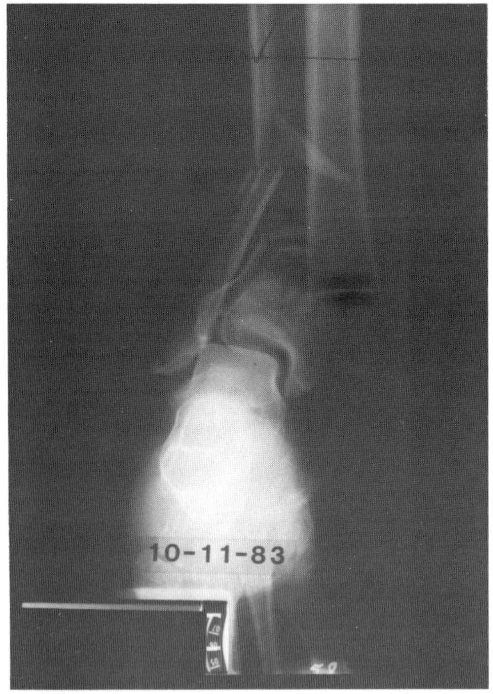

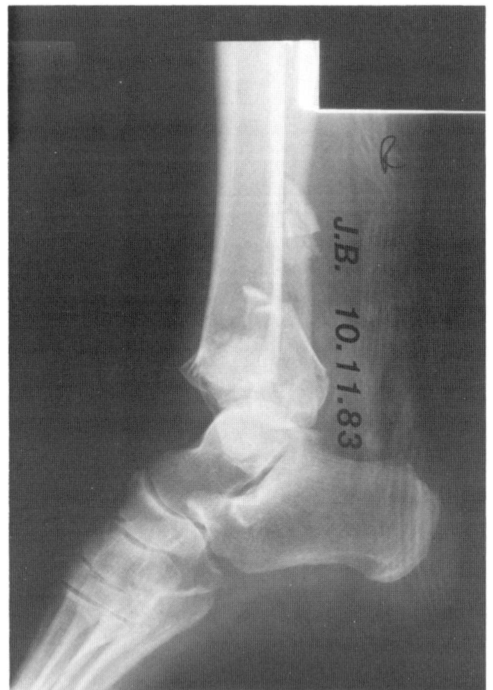

A

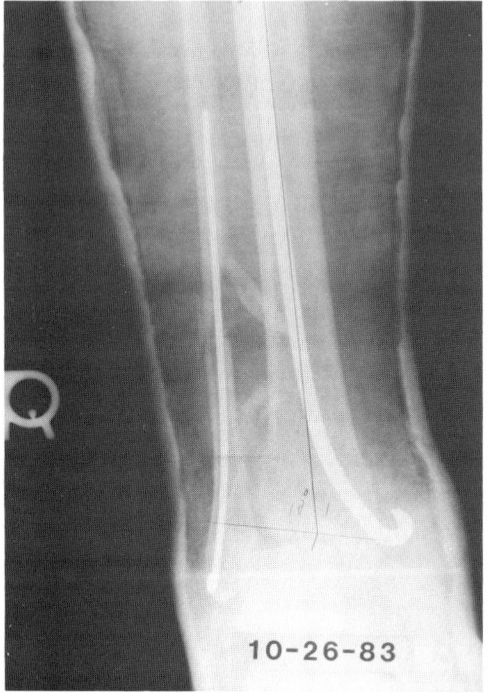

B

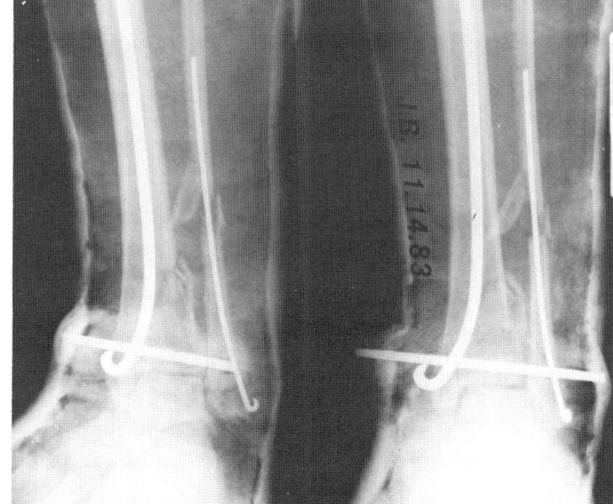

C

Figure 10–12. (**A**) On October 11, 1983, a comminuted supramalleolar fracture with a more proximal fracture of the fibula was treated by Dr. John Reynolds, with a ³⁄₃₂-inch (2.38 mm) fibular pin and a (4.76 mm) dynamic pin from the medial distal aspect of the tibia. (**B**) The limb was placed in a cast and at 13 days after fixation it was noticed that the tibial plafond was going into 10-degree valgus tilt. (**C**) The patient was returned to surgery (continued)

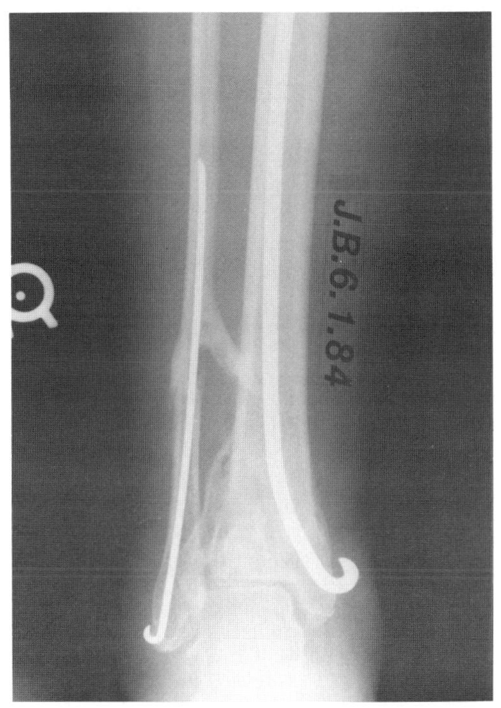

D

Figure 10–12 (cont.).   during which a Steinmann pin was inserted parallel to the plafond and
external fixation was used in addition to the Rush
pin fixation, giving a brilliant result on November
14, 1983. (D) After the fracture started to consoli-
date, the external fixation pin was removed and the
patient was started on active range of motion. The
plafond showed a normal position on June 6, 1984.
(E) On July 27, 1984, the pins were removed on an
outpatient basis. These radiographs show absence
of fracture disease.

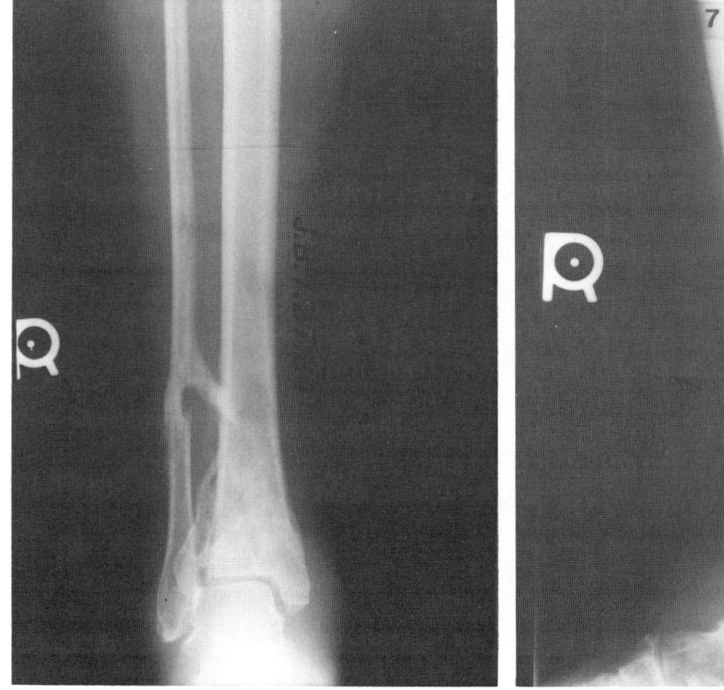

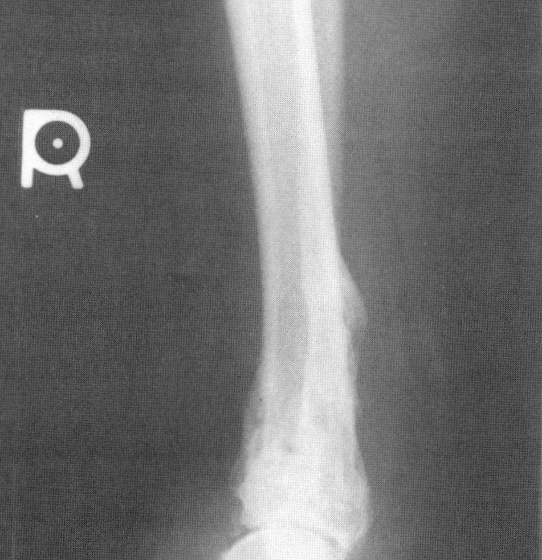

E

REFERENCES

1. Ashurst, A.P.C., Bromer, R.S.: Classification and mechanism of fracture of the leg bones involving the ankle. Arch. Surg. 4:51–129, 1922.
2. Laüge-Hansen, N.: Fractures of the ankle. Arch. Surg. 56:259–317, 1948.
3. Mueller, M.E., Allgower, M., Schneider, R., Willenegger, H.: Manual of Internal Fixation. New York, Springer, Second edition, expanded and revised, 1979. p. 288–289, 1979.
4. Yablon, I.G., Heller, F.G., House, S., Leroy, A. The key role of the lateral malleolus in displaced fractures of the ankle. J. Bone Joint Surg. 59A:169–173, 1977.
5. Leach, R.E.: A means of stabilizing comminuted distal tibial fractures. J. Trauma 4:722–726, 1964.

SUGGESTED READINGS

Rush, L.V.: Atlas of Rush Pin Technics. Meridian, Mississippi, The Berivon Company, 1955.

CHAPTER 11

Fractures in Conjunction with Metal Implants

Acute Femoral Shaft Fractures with Uncemented Austin-Moore Hip
    Prostheses
Acute Femoral Shaft Fractures with Healed, Internally Fixed Hip Fractures
Acute Ipsilateral Hip and Femur Shaft Fractures
Supracondylar Femur Fractures with a Total Knee Prosthesis
Acute Shaft Fractures with Retained Screws

Implants that traverse the medullary canal longitudinally or by transverse screws may be fixed with intramedullary pins by passing the screws or paralleling the implant. The femur is the most frequently injured bone that may have prosthetic implants at either end of the shaft, and most of the discussion concerns the femur.

ACUTE FRACTURES OF THE FEMORAL SHAFT WITH UNCEMENTED AUSTIN-MOORE HIP PROSTHESES

Acute fractures of the femoral shaft about a uncemented Austin-Moore prosthesis are usually spiral in nature. The spiral fractures require retubulation with cerclage wire while the pin, either a ¼-inch (6.35 mm) or a ³⁄₁₆-inch (4.76 mm), is inserted next to the prosthesis from the proximal end. The pin is easily placed in the anterolateral border of the femur adjacent to the prosthesis. The pin can be placed next to the prosthesis at the tip of the trochanter, but better rotational control is possible from the anterolateral aspect of the trochanter. The pin is only slightly prebent (Fig. 11–1).

Cerclage wires are wrapped around the spiral fracture first, and then the pin is put down to the level of the top of the patella (Fig. 11–2).

Acute Fractures of the Femoral Shaft with Healed, Internally Fixed Fractures at the Hip

Acute fractures of the femoral neck can be treated early with Knowles pins or with a sliding hip screw and still the shaft of the femur can be fixed by passage of a pin between the screws from the greater trochanter area down to the distal third of

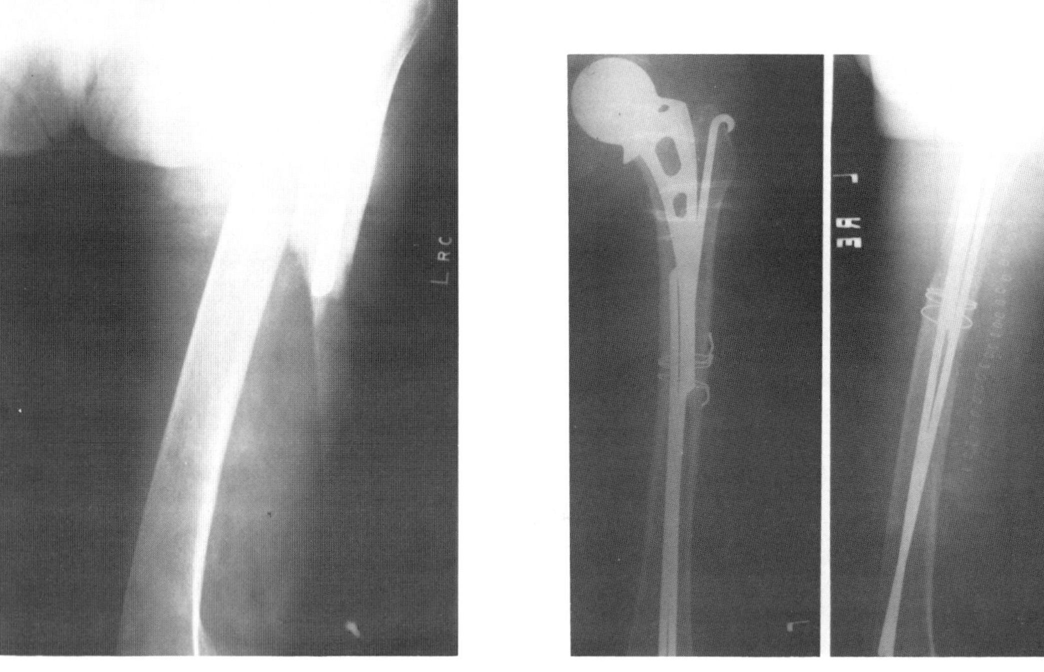

A   B

Figure 11–1. Acute fractures of the femoral shaft with Hip endoprosthesis. (**A**) An 89-year-old woman with a previous successful Austin-Moore prosthesis slipped, suffering a spiral fracture in the distal inch of the femur at the level of the tip of the prosthesis. (**B**) The patient was placed on the fracture table, the fracture was aligned, two cerclage wires were passed to hold the fracture, and then a ³⁄₁₆-inch (4.76 mm) pin was passed from the greater trochanter across the fracture site and a second pin placed from the lateral femoral condyle. This provided firm fixation, and the patient was again walking with a walker.

the femur for stability. If there is difficulty in getting by one of the screws, the screw could, of course, be removed, since the femoral fracture is already healed (Fig. 11–3).

CONCOMITANT IPSILATERAL FRACTURES AT THE HIP AND OF THE FEMORAL SHAFT

Concomitant ipsilateral fractures of the femoral shaft and at the hip are uncommon but have been treated with various methods of internal fixation such as Knowles pins or sliding hip screws. The caveat for the slide plate and screw fixation is to put the screws as divergent as possible so that there is a triangular area

through which a longitudinal pin can be directed (Fig. 11–4).

SUPRACONDYLAR FRACTURES WITH TOTAL KNEE ARTHROPLASTY

Supracondylar fractures with total knee replacement arthroplasty occur more frequently, and fixation is difficult by most means (Fig. 11–5). Fixation with plates is not usually successful, and traction for final treatment is advised but takes many weeks and may result in joint stiffness. The technique is the same as that for fresh supracondylar fractures. However, the location of the awl reamer hole is critical and must be at a point on the

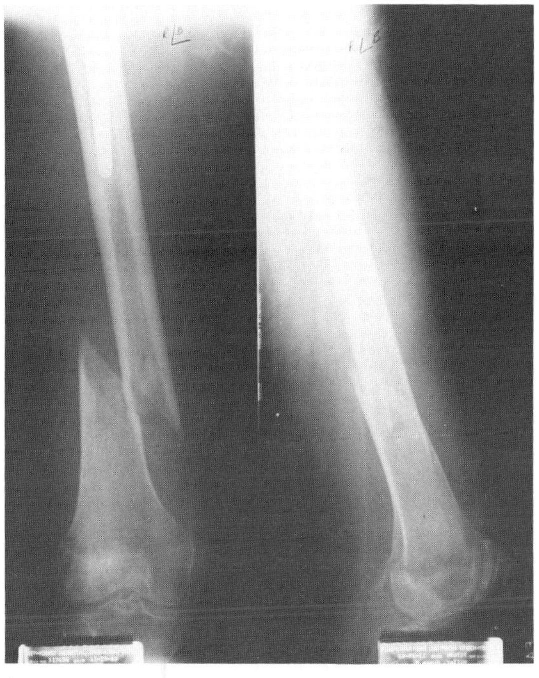 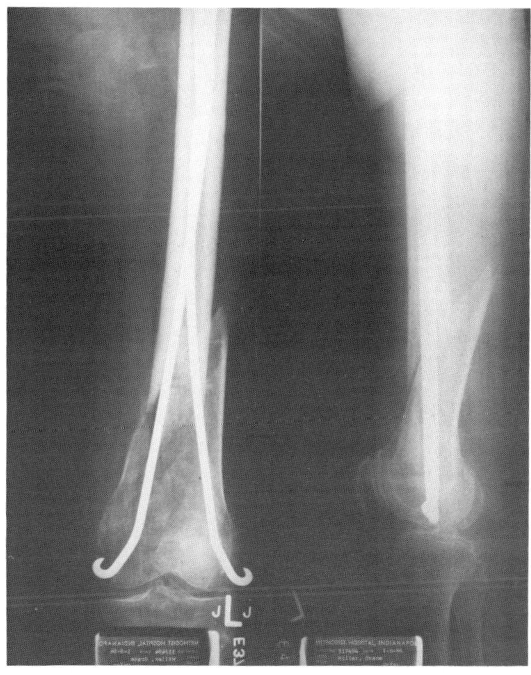

A
B

Figure 11–2.   (A) A 67-year-old woman with a Thompson hip prosthesis slipped and fell in 1963, sustaining an oblique, slightly comminuted fracture at the distal end of the femoral shaft. (B) This was reduced inadequately on the regular operating table with the use of a knee rest and two ³⁄₁₆-inch (4.76 mm) pins were placed across the fracture proximally to entwine the prosthesis. Now better treatment would be obtained with the use of a single cerclage wire and the use of the fracture table with an image intensifier.

medial and lateral sides in line with the center of the proximal part of the femoral shaft. Great care should be taken in the reduction of the fracture, particularly in the lateral view, so that the straight ³⁄₁₆-inch (4.76 mm) pins are inserted across the fracture and develop a dynamic bending by bouncing off the proximal part of the medullary canal. Placement of the awl reamer hole in the center of the C of the metallic femoral prosthesis will result in recurvatum of the total knee prosthesis, and function will be impaired (Figs. 11–6, 11–7).

Remember, a stiff knee transmits more stress to the fracture site and slow healing is frequent. Early motion for the supracondylar fracture in a leg with a previously normal total knee prosthesis is still important.

FRACTURE OF THE FEMORAL SHAFT WITH SCREWS TRANSVERSING THE SHAFT

For the fractured femoral shaft with screws that transverse it the screw usually does not need to be removed, as most of the time a ¼-inch (6.35 mm) pin, with the sled runner tip helping the pin pass by the medullary screw, allows for fixation of the fracture without removing the medullary impediment (Fig. 11–8).

SUGGESTED READING

Rush, L.V.: Atlas of Rush Pin Technics. Meridian, Mississippi, The Berivon Company, 1955.

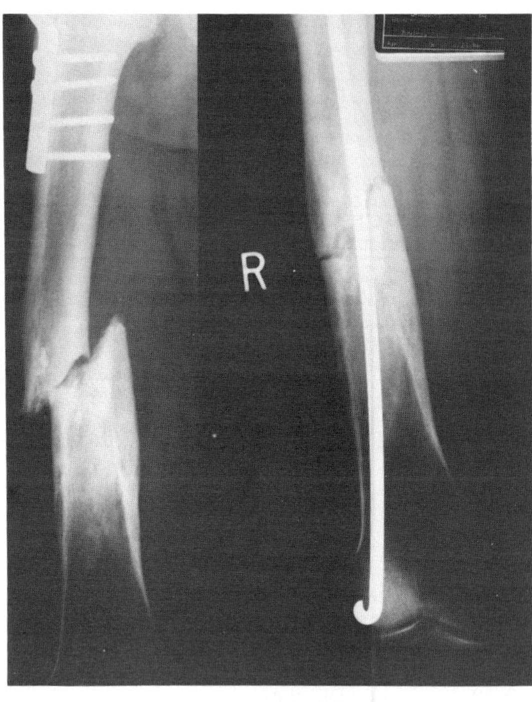

A

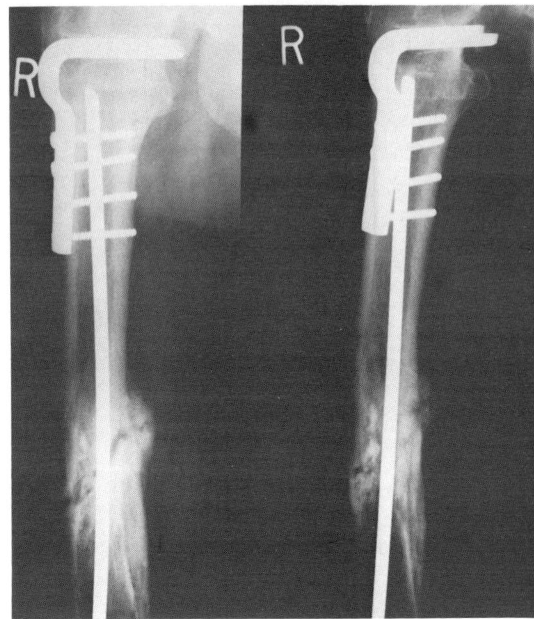

B

Figure 11–3. (**A**) A 32-year-old male schoolteacher previously had had an open fracture as a teenager, involving the right femoral shaft, and had been placed in traction at the time. He developed some osteoarthritis in his hip, and a hip osteotomy was performed in 1982 for the arthritis. While playing baseball on July 19, 1986, he suffered an oblique fracture through the same area of his previous open fracture. (**B**) The patient was taken to surgery and on the fracture table with an image intensifier, a ¼-inch (6.35 mm) pin was inserted from the lateral femoral condyle across the fracture closed and past the four AO screws in the osteotomy plate. The patient used crutches, the fracture healed to painless weight-bearing, and he was teaching school by October 20, 1986.

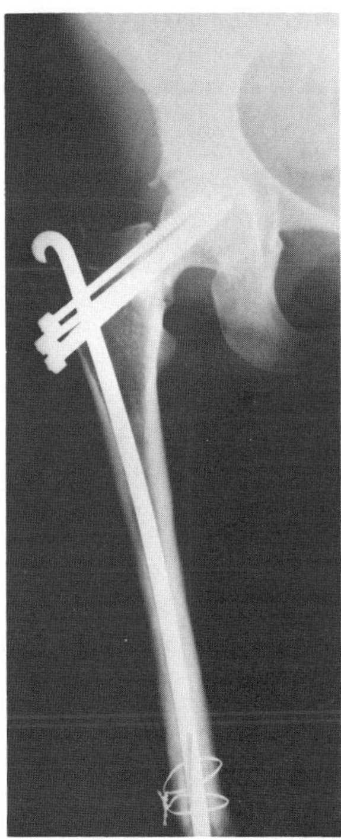

Figure 11–4. Ipsilateral fracture at the hip and of the shaft. In March 1979 a 26-year-old woman suffered polytrauma with a segmental femoral fracture, displaced femoral neck fracture, and a compression fracture of the second and third lumbar vertebrae. Within 24 hours, she was taken to surgery where the fracture was reduced on the fracture table. The hip was exposed and four Knowles pins were inserted at the fracture site using the image intensifier. A precurved ¼-inch (6.35 mm) Rush pin was passed between the Knowles pins to the fracture in the distal end of the shaft where the cerclage wires were then tightened and the pin seated into the lateral femoral condyle. Both the femoral neck fracture and the femoral shaft fracture proceeded to healing and as of July 1981 radiographs showed no signs of avascular necrosis of the head of the femur.

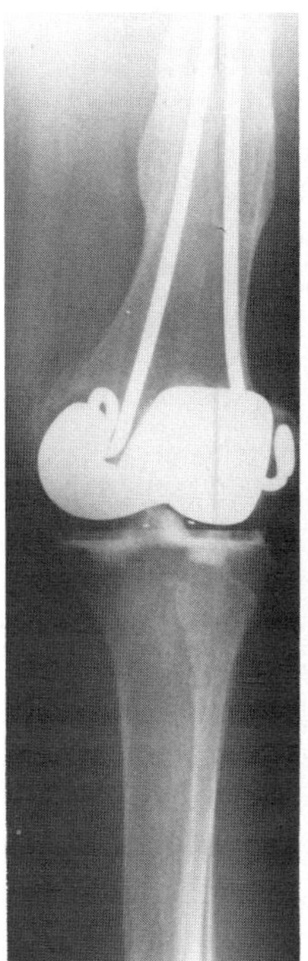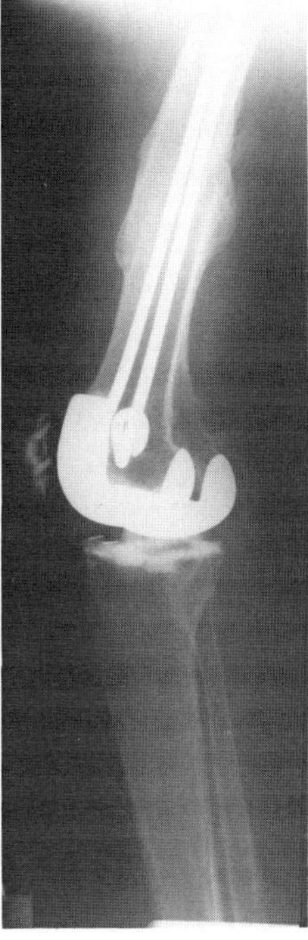

Figure 11–5. Fractures proximal to a total knee prosthesis. A 61-year-old woman 1½ years after a total knee arthroplasty, suffered a fall at home with a displaced fracture at the distal end of the femoral shaft. After closed reduction on the fracture table, two straight looped condylar pins were inserted across the fracture site, in a surgical time of 35 minutes. Active knee motion was started and the patient was healed with full weight-bearing at 7 months.

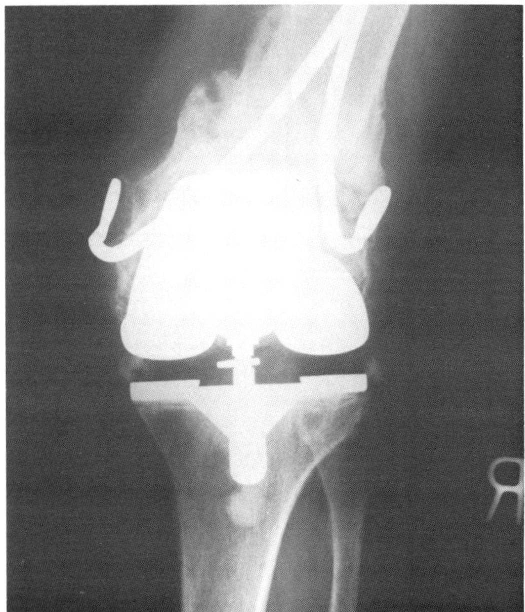
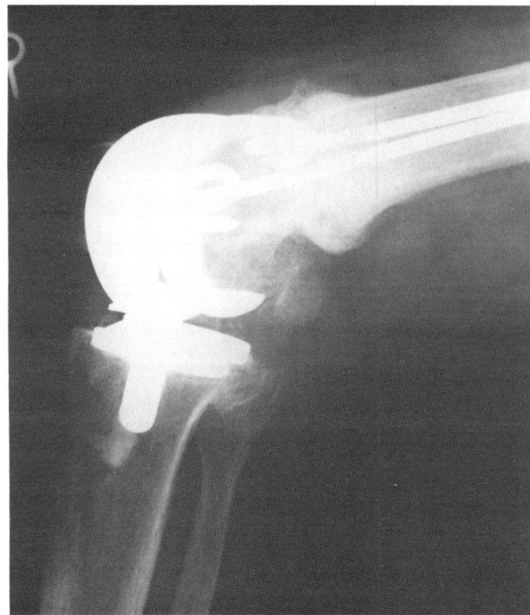

Figure 11–6. A 56-year-old woman with rheumatoid arthritis and a total knee prosthesis suffered a supracondylar fracture after a mild fall. The fracture was not well reduced on the fracture table, and the pins were inserted too proximally. Only the lateral pin was stress relieved, leaving a mild valgus deformity at healing. Early active motion was encouraged.

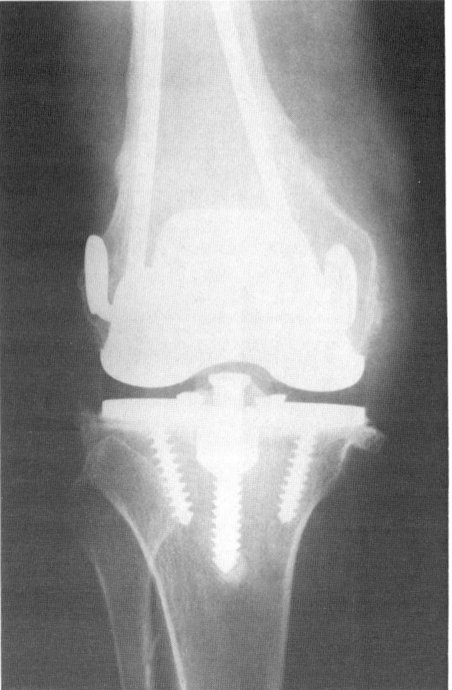
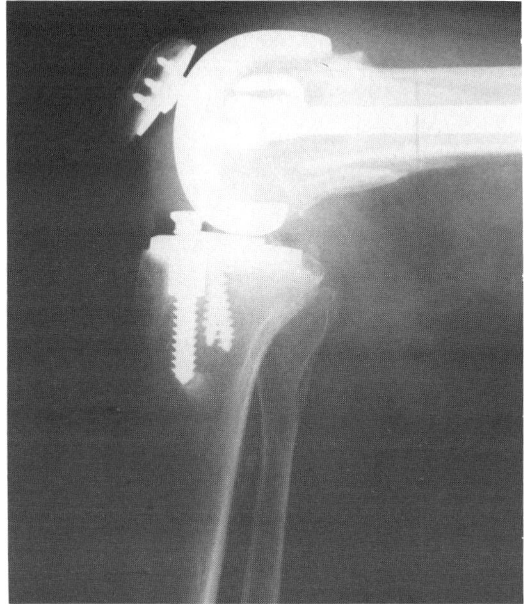

Figure 11–7. A 72-year-old woman suffered a supracondylar fracture that was pinned with looped condylar pins 4 months before she returned to surgery for a total knee replacement arthroplasty. This was done without removing the looped condylar pins and using a short intramedullary guide for the femoral prosthesis cutting jigs. The patient proceeded to a range of motion of 0 to 114 degrees.

114

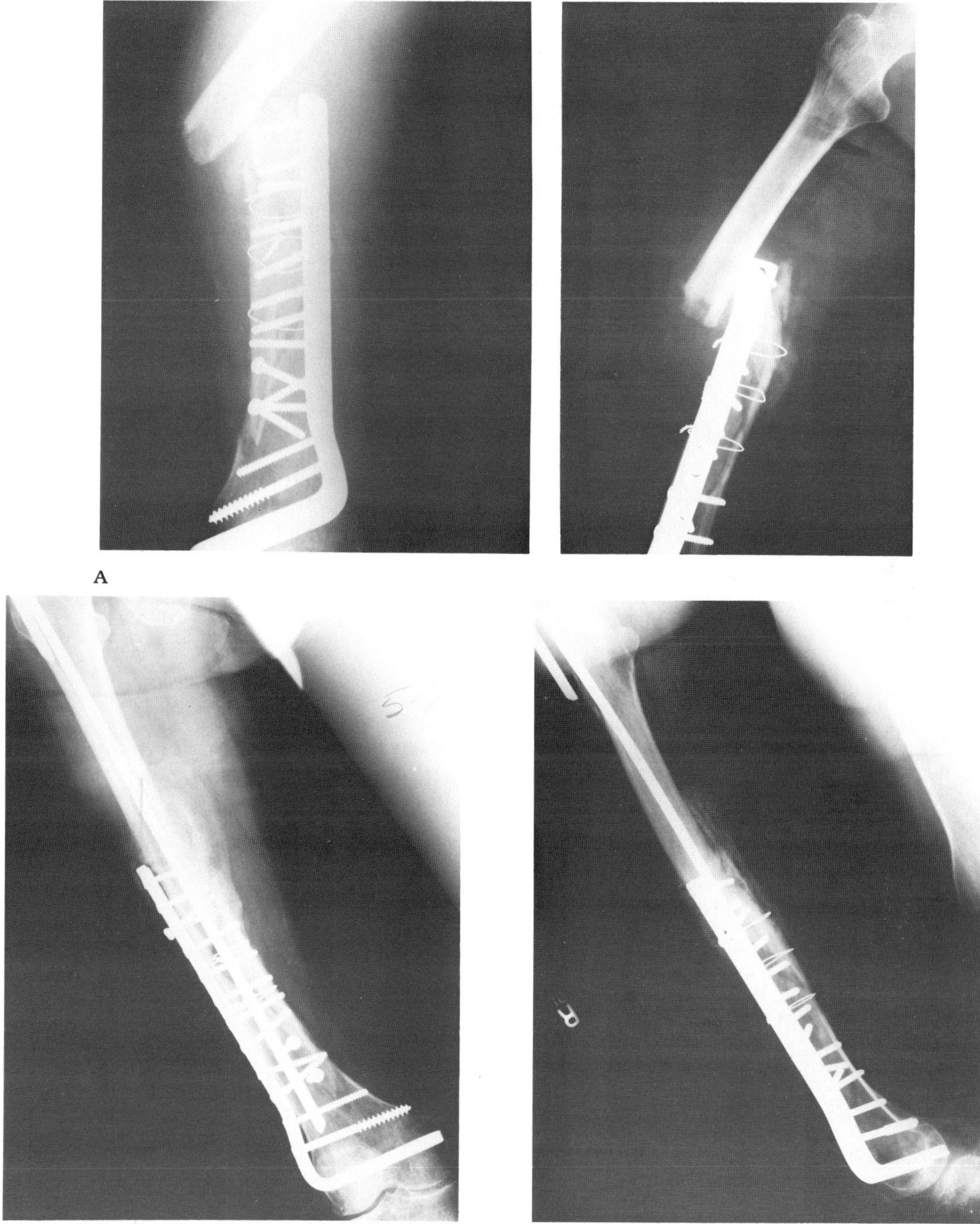

Figure 11–8. Fracture of the femoral shaft with screws transversing the shaft. (**A**) A 70-year-old woman had a comminuted displaced fracture in the distal third of the femur treated with an 11 hole supracondylar plate months before she slipped and suffered a displaced fracture at the proximal end on April 13, 1989. (**B**) The patient was taken to surgery and a precurved shepherd's crook Rush pin was passed from the greater trochanter past 12 screws into the distal end of the femur without opening the fracture site. By May 27, 1988, the patient was healed and weight-bearing. The pin was passed by the screws by rotating the head of the pin to allow the sled runner to slide past the transverse screws.

CHAPTER 12

Fracture Care in the Patient with Multiple System Trauma

Immediate Stabilization of Fractures in Patients with Multiple System Trauma
The Floating Knee
Bilateral Femur Fractures

A patient with polytrauma is defined as one who:

1. Has an unstable fracture or fractures, dislocation of a major bone, the pelvis or spine;
2. Has suffered high-energy blunt trauma;
3. Has injured two organ systems or more, each having an abbreviated injury score (AIS-85) of 3 or more;
4. Has an Injury Severity Score of over 25.

Patients with polytrauma die in the first 24 hours primarily from severe head injury or uncontrolled hemorrhage, in the first 7 to 10 days from an adult respiratory distress syndrome (ARDS), and after 10 days from multiple system organ failure. Approximately 30 percent of the patients with an ISS score of higher than 20 who have femoral fractures treated by skeletal traction will die from ARDS or multiple system organ failure. Immediate fixation of fractures of the long bones and

pelvis greatly reduces this and makes treatment of other injuries more simple.

IMMEDIATE STABILIZATION OF FRACTURES

A trauma patient presents unique problems in the planning of acute care which involves a multidisciplinary approach. An excellent plan, described by Meyers[1] in his excellent text, *The Multiply Injured Patient with Complex Fractures*, is in five stages:[1]

1. Resuscitation
2. Phase of immediate operation—usually threatening hemorrhage
3. Phase of stabilization
4. Stage of delayed operative procedures
5. Phase of recovery

The phase of delayed operative procedure is where the orthopaedic trauma team fits in. Many times phases 2, 3, and

116

4 are concurrent. Riska and colleagues[2] advocated primary operative fixation of long bone fractures in patients with multiple trauma. Chapman[3] has written extensively on this, and we have done this in the Indiana series for a number of years.

THE FLOATING KNEE

The floating knee is an ipsilateral fracture of the tibial and femoral shaft. These are complete fractures and require attention in the patient with multiple trauma. The ideal position for surgery is supine, as the general, chest, neurologic, and urologic surgeons are more comfortable operating with the patient in this position. Simultaneous surgery can be done on the extension fracture table with the knee rest and the image intensifier. Entrance to the femoral medullary canal and the tibia can easily be made with the awl reamer from the medial or lateral side of the femur and tibia, respectively, at the knee, and the fractures can be treated without any undue problem. If blood loss is a problem, a tourniquet can be placed in the proximal part of the thigh to preserve blood at this time (Fig. 12–1).

The two-pin technique for the proximal part of the tibia, tibial shaft, and distal part of the tibia as well as for the distal part of the femur can easily be done. The technique using a single ¼-inch (6.35 mm) pin for the femoral shaft has been described previously (Fig. 12–2).

BILATERAL FRACTURES OF THE FEMORAL SHAFT

I have made an offset knee rest for the Rush table for both femurs for pinning fractures in the supine position. Image intensification in anteroposterior views can be done with ease, and the lateral views are easy to differentiate because of the angle difference in the femurs.

Reduction by closed methods is advantageous using traction, crutch and strap, or femoral wrench as mentioned previously, but is best done prior to the surgical preparation of the skin. A precurved pin will allow reduction of segmental fractures that are too difficult to be reduced by purely closed techniques (Fig. 12–3).

The simplicity of the semi-open technique must take precedence over the urge to do all of the surgery by closed method. I have seen no difference in healing or infection rates of fractures treated with the semi-open technique (Fig. 12–4).

SEGMENTAL FRACTURES

The use of a precurved ¼-inch (6.35 mm) pin will allow reduction of segmental fractures that are too difficult to be reduced with standard closed techniques. Rapid effective surgery should get the multiply injured patient into the phase of recovery with the least delay.

REFERENCES

1. Claudi, B.F., Meyers M.H., eds.: Priorities in the Treatment of the multiply Injured Patient with musculoskeletal Injuries. "The Multiply Injured Patient with Complex Fractures." M.H. Meyers. Philadelphia, Lea and Febiger, Chapter 1, p. 4.
2. Riska, E.B., von Bonsdorff, H., Hakkinen S., et al.: Primary operative fixation of long bone fractures in patients with multiple injuries. J. Trauma 17:111–121, 1977.
3. Chapman, M.W.: The use of immediate internal fixation in open fractures. Orthop. Clin. North Am. 11:579–591, 1980.

SUGGESTED READINGS

Beam, H.P., Jr., Seligson, N.: Nine cases of bilateral femoral shaft fractures: a composite view. J. Trauma 20:399–402, 1980.

Figure 12–1.   Floating knee. **(A)** In 1978, a 20-year-old man was in an automobile accident at college and suffered a displaced intracondylar Y and supracondylar fracture of the femur, a fracture of the tibia at the junction of the middle and distal third, and cerebral concussion. The femoral fracture was reduced on the fracture table prior to skin preparation and observation with the image intensifier confirmed the reduction. Radiographs of the femur. **(B)** The tibia was internally fixed through the same skin preparation at the knee with a precurved ¼-inch (6.35 mm) pin going into the distal end. Active motion was started on crutches. The femur healed in 12 weeks and the tibia in 20 weeks. Range of motion at the knee was 0 to 140 degrees at the time of pin removal, at approximately 1 year. Radiographs of the tibia.

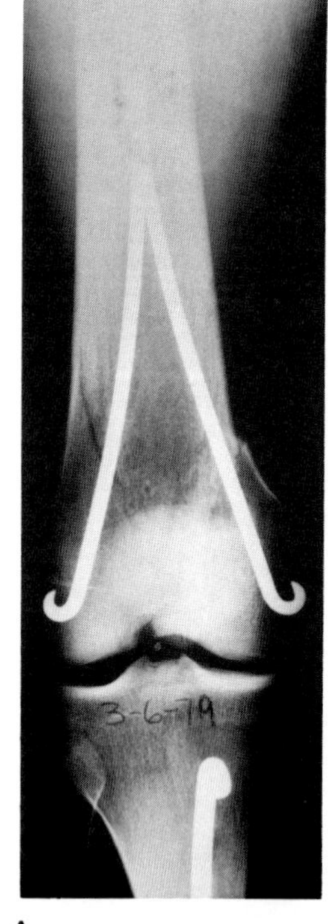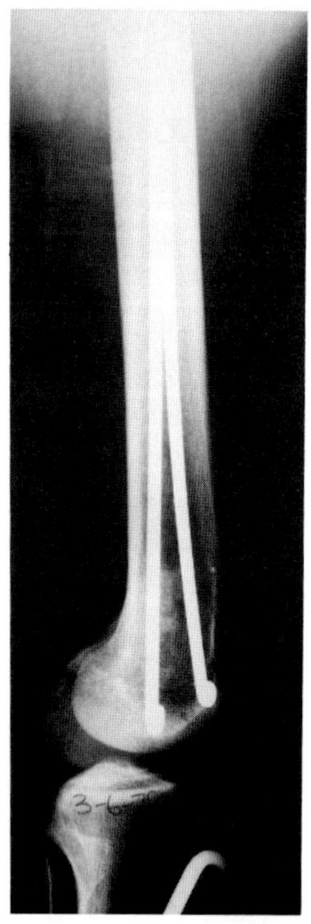

A

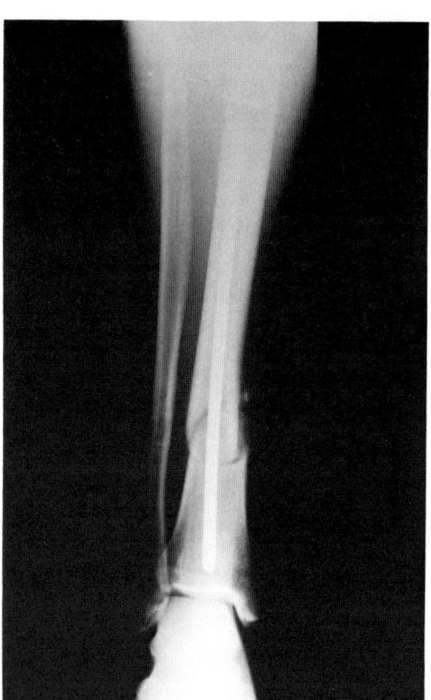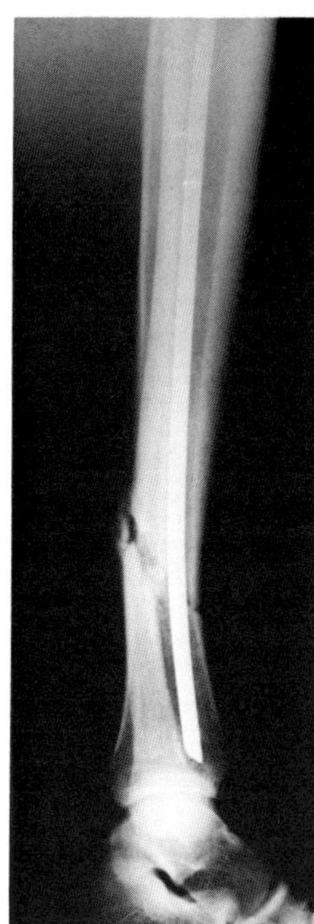

B

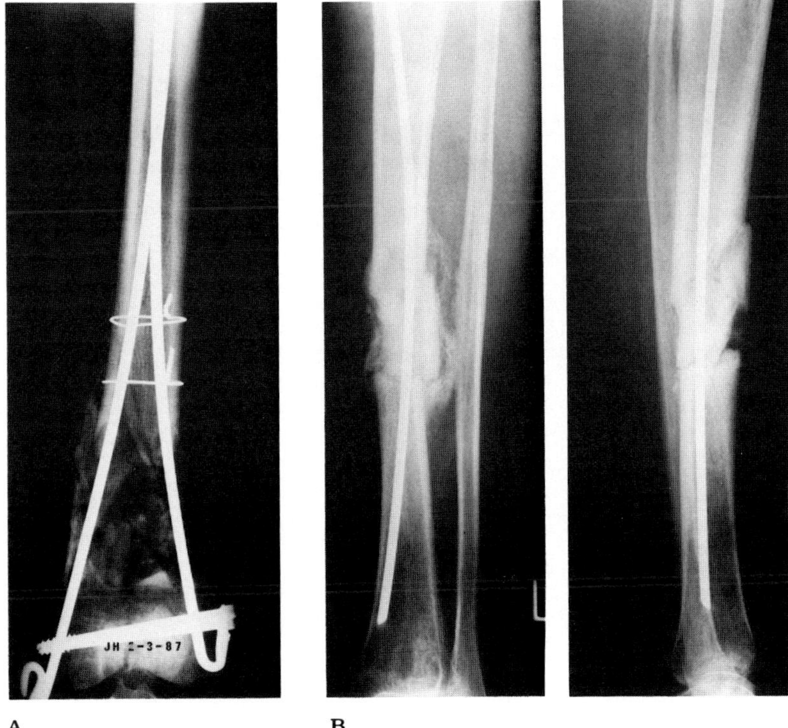

Figure 12–2.   (A) A male had a floating knee due to a comminuted supracondylar fracture in the distal end of the femur, and a comminuted tibial shaft fracture. The fracture was reduced on the Rush table with a knee rest, before skin preparation of the thigh and leg. Cerclage wires were placed around the femoral shaft first and then straight looped condylar pins were inserted into the proximal part of the femur. At the end of this surgery, two AO screws were placed through the knee incisions. **(B)** A third incision at the knee was made for insertion of a ³⁄₁₆-inch (4.76 mm) precurved Rush pin. Knee motion was initiated at 10 days. The femoral fracture was healed in 4 months, and the tibia was healed in 7 months.

Bone, L.B., Bucholz, R.: The management of fractures in the patient with multiple trauma. J. Bone Joint Srg. 68A:945–949, 1986.

Johnson, D., Cadombi, A., Burton, S.G.: Incidence of adult respiratory distress syndrome in patients with multiple musculoskeletal injuries: effect of early stabilization of fractures. J. Trauma 25:375–384, 1985.

Ram, A.: Bilateral floating knees in a multiply injured patient. Orthopedics 9:1355–1358, 1986.

Rush, L.V.: Atlas of Rush Pin Technics. Meridian, Mississippi, The Berivon Company, 1955.

Winquist, R.A.: Segmental fractures of the lower extremity and the floating knee. The Multiply Injured Patient with Complex Fractures, edited by Meyers, M.H. Philadelphia, Lea and Febiger, p. 218–248, 1984.

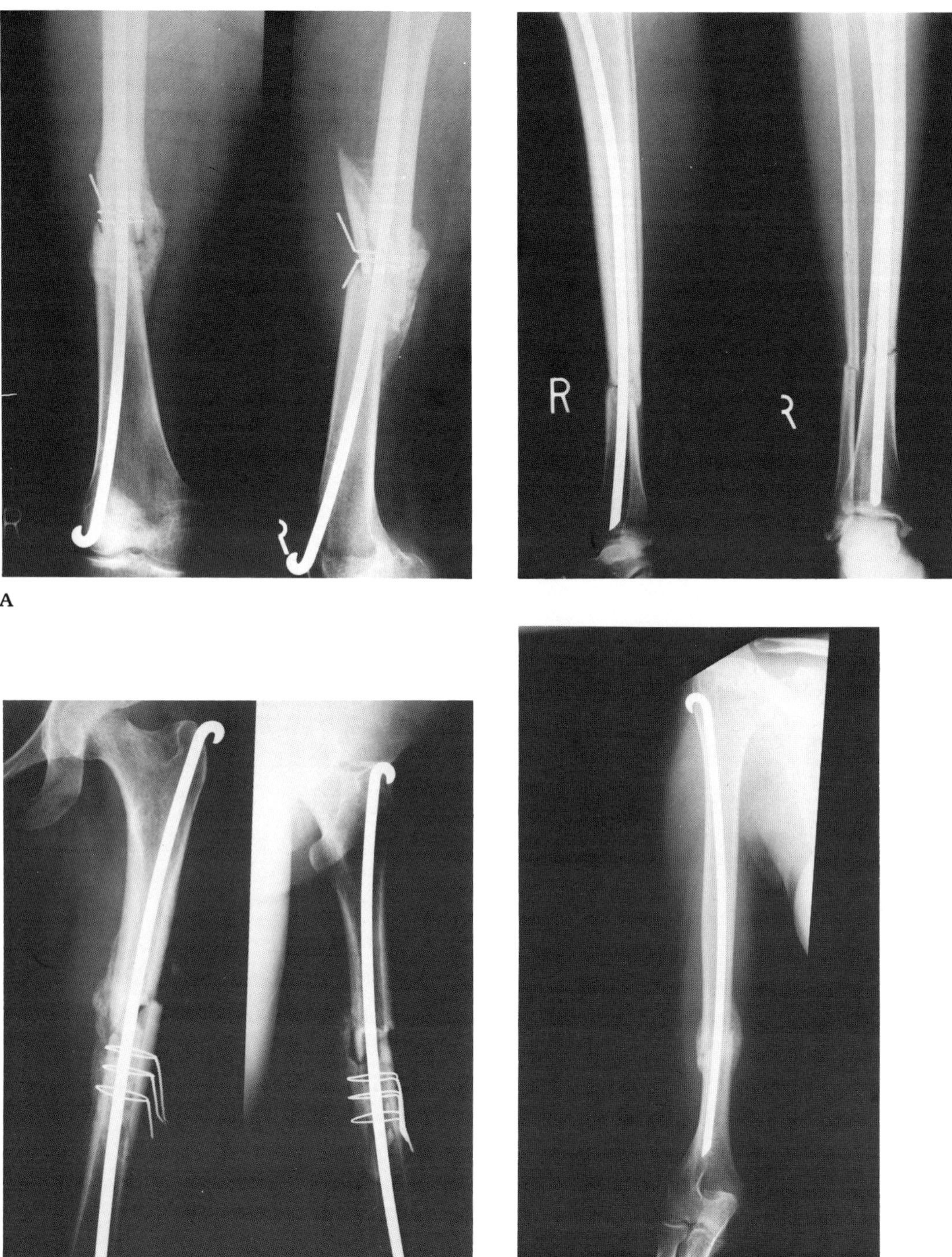

Figure 12–3.   Bilateral fractures of the femoral shaft (**A**) A 22-year-old woman had polytrauma in April 1988 with a right open Gustilo Grade II fracture, as well as fractures of the right tibia and right humerus. Please see Chapter 7 for treatment of the humeral fracture. The right femur and tibia are shown here. (**B**) The patient was taken to surgery within 24 hours after injury and placed on the Rush fracture table with the special bilateral countersupports for the knee and one image intensifier. Two surgeons were used to pin the open femoral fracture and the closed left femoral and right tibial fractures simultaneously. The left femur is shown here. (**C**) The humeral fracture was healed by June 22, and the femurs were started on assisted weight-bearing by July 18, 1988.

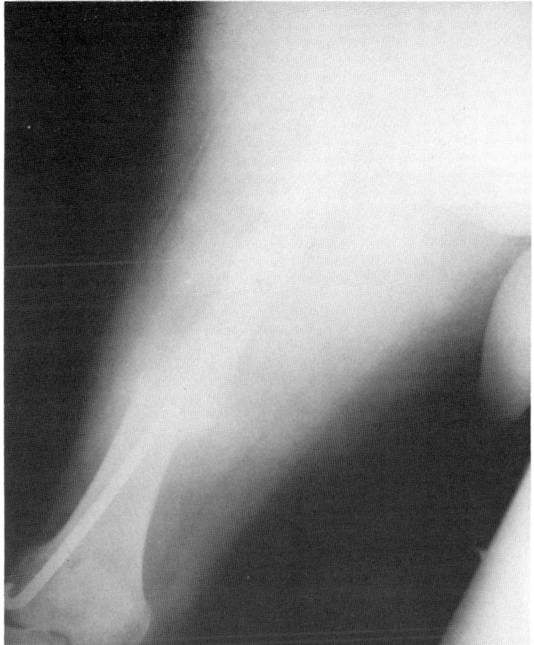

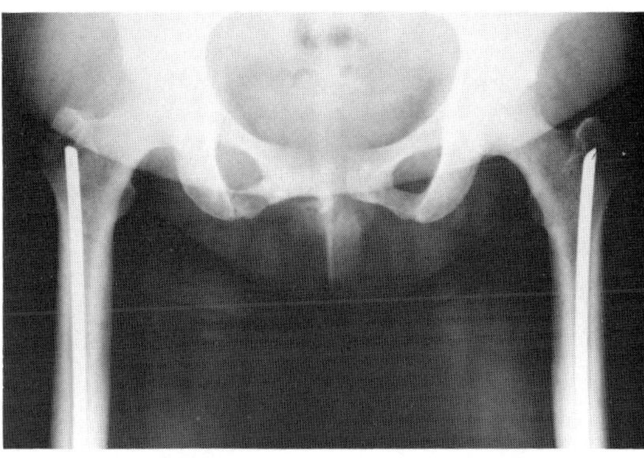

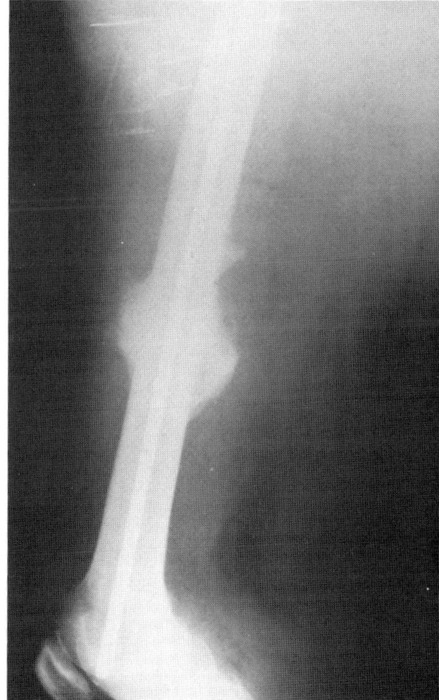

Figure 12–4. A 56-year-old hypertensive woman who was considerably obese was in a car and truck accident and had surgery on the day of the injury. Bilateral closed pinnings were done in the femur at one anesthetic session, but because of only a single unilateral countersupport, reduction and pinning were done separately. Both fractures healed in 5 months.

CHAPTER 13

Treatment of Open Fractures

Debridement
Antibiotic Treatment
Atraumatic Pinning to Provide Stability
Secondary Wound Closure
Return to Function

As noted by Gustilo and Anderson in 1976,[1] the most important prognostic factor in open fractures is the level of injury producing the wound and thus the extent of the soft-tissue injury. The corollary and the next most prognostic factor in open fracture is the level of surgical trauma necessary to stabilize the injured tissues by effective immobilization of the fracture. In the atlas published in 1955, Leslie Rush said, "Pinning is almost routinely indicated in fresh compound fractures, not only to maintain the bone reconstruction but to mitigate against infection."[2] The marrow cavity is much less susceptible to infection than previously believed.[3] The pin is an asset if infection occurs before final healing.

CLASSIFICATION OF OPEN FRACTURES[4]

Types

I.   Open Fractures with a Wound Less Than 1 cm (¼ inch) Long and Clean

II. Open Fractures With a Laceration More than 2 cm (½ inch) Without Extensive Soft-tissue Damage, Flaps, or Avulsion

III. Either an Open Segmental Fracture or Open Fracture with Extensive Soft-Tissue Damage or a Traumatic Amputation

A.   Shotgun Wounds

B.   Open Fractures Caused by a Farm Injury

C.   Any Open Fracture Accompanying Vascular Injury Requiring Repair

Sterile metal in a potentially infected wound is not a cause of infection. Sterile metal performing a function is different. It stabilizes the bones and fortunately stabilizes the traumatized soft tissues. "Once infection occurs, the presence of an implant is advantageous as long as it provides stability," wrote Rittmann and colleagues in 1978 (Figs. 13–1, 13–2).

The basic tenants of treatment are:

1. Immediate adequate debridement and irrigation, repeat debridement and irrigation of all Type III open fractures,

122

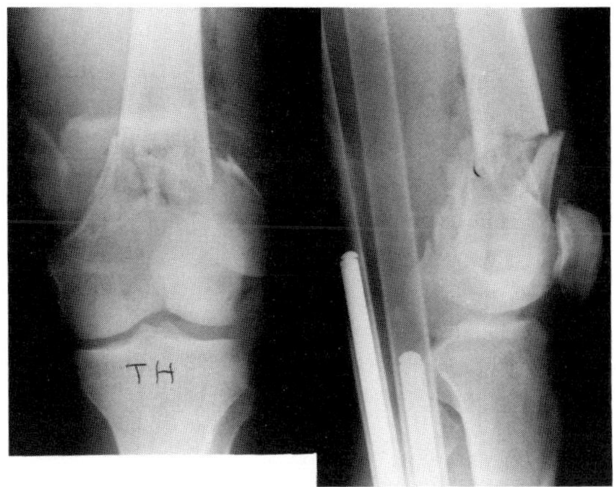

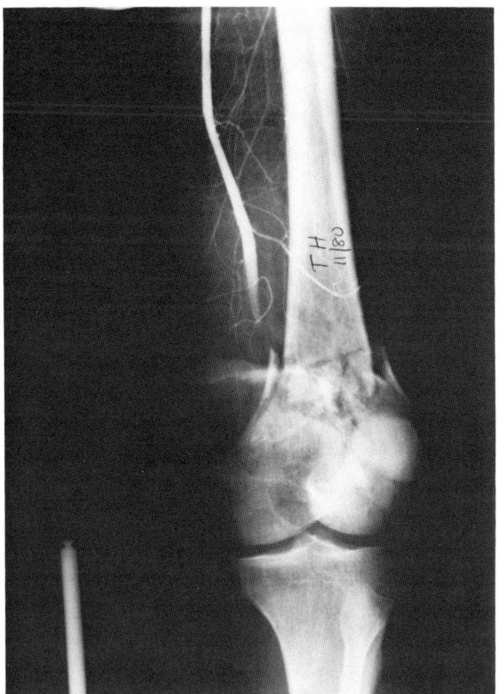

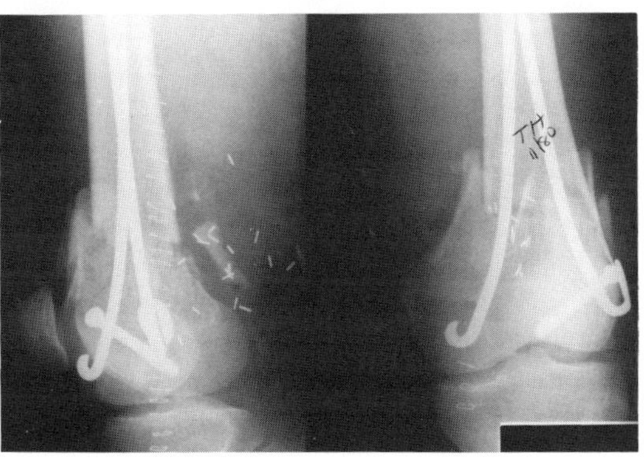

Figure 13–1. A 22-year-old man had a motorcycle injury, with a Gustilo Type IIIC comminuted supracondylar fracture as well as an anterolateral condylar fracture. The femur was pinned prior to vascular repair in November 1980. The arterial repair was successful, and the fracture progressed to healing.

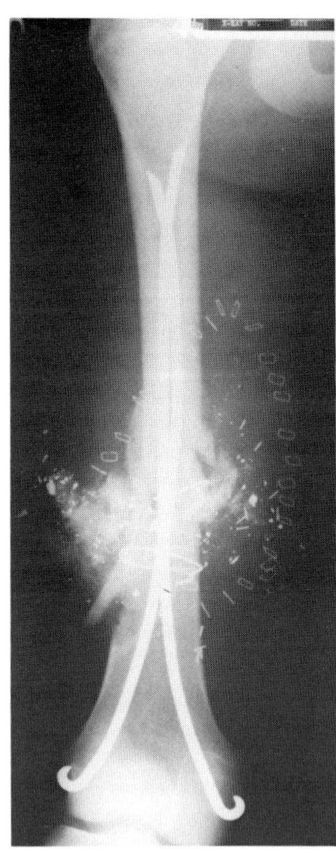

Figure 13–2. A 20-year-old man had a gunshot wound with a Gustilo Type IIIC comminuted fracture in the distal part of the shaft with arterial laceration. The wound was debrided. Two ³⁄₁₆-inch (4.76 mm) pins were used with cerclage wire, and the arterial repair carried out. The pins were precariously long. No infection occurred postoperatively.

and retaining large bone fragments for stability

2. Appropriate antibiotic therapy
3. Securing effective fracture stability
4. Wound coverage. The goal of soft-tissue coverage within 5 to 10 days. Delayed primary closure (DPC) for type I and II with skin graft, local flaps, or microvascular transfer in Type III fractures
5. Early cancellous bone grafting after wound healing
6. Deciding on early amputation

My expertise with Rush pin fixation in open fractures has gradually increased with experience. All are now treated with internal fixation with Rush pins; all Type II and Type III fractures are left open and scheduled for redebridement or DPC in a few days. Patients in Type IIIB and IIIC group are returned for re-debridement earlier than Type II or IIIA. Type I is left open (Figs. 13–3, 13–4).

A critical review of early infections, following immediate internal fixation in open fractures, revealed that the cause of infection is mainly due to repeated mistakes including disregard of the basic principles of soft-tissue handling, poor knowledge of appropriate instrumentation, improper application of adequate implants, and finally, limited technical skills due to the lack of significant experience with open fractures.[6]

REFERENCES

1. Gustilo, R.B., Anderson, J.T.: Prevention of infection in treatment of one thousand and twenty five open fractures of long bones. J. Bone Joint Surg. 58A:453–458, 1976.
2. Rush, L.V.: Atlas of Rush Pin Technics. Meridian, Mississippi, The Berivon Company, p. 80, 1955.
3. Rush, H.L., Jr., Fitts, W.T., Gibbons, J., Monroe, E.W.: Intramedullary nailing in the presence of infection. An experimental study in dogs. Surg. Gynecol. Obstet. 94:727–732, 1952.
4. Gustilo, R.B.: Management of Open Fractures and Their Complications. Vol. IV. Saunders Monographs in Clinical Orthopaedics. Philadelphia, W.B. Saunders, 1982.
5. Rittmann, W.W., Scheble, M., Matter, P., Allgower, M.: Open fractures: long-term results in two hundred consecutive cases. Clin. Ortho. 138:132–140, 1978.
6. Claudi, B.F., Meyers, M.H., eds.: Priorities in the treatment of the multiply injured patient with musculoskeletal injuries. "The Multiply Injured Patient with Complex Fractures." M.H. Meyers. Philadelphia, Lea and Febiger, p. 7, 1984.

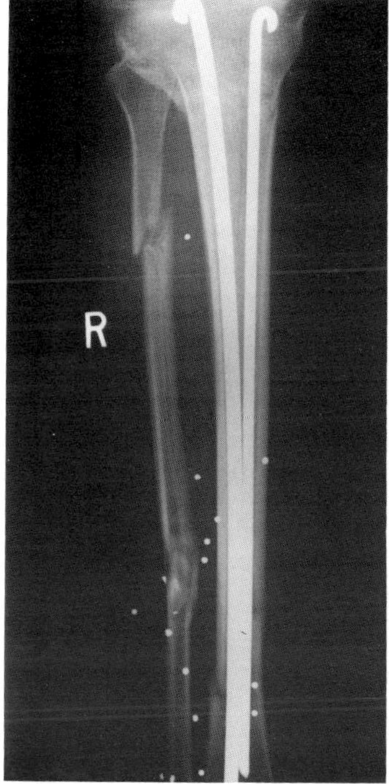
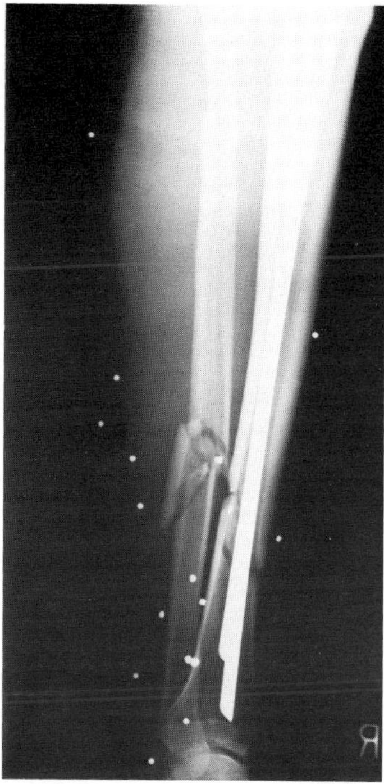

A

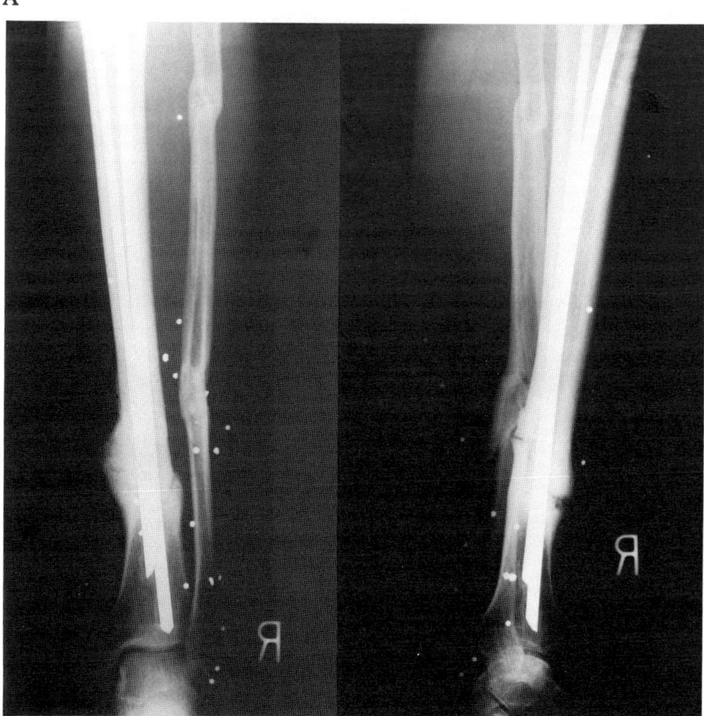

B

Figure 13–3. Open tibial fracture. (**A**) A 37-year-old accident victim had a Gustilo Type III fracture of the distal aspect of the tibia and fracture of the proximal aspect that was closed. The buckshot pellets are from a previous injury. The patient was debrided on the fracture table, and two pins were inserted close to the tibial articular surface and down into the distal end, with the pins covering both fractures. Delayed closure was done for the open wound. (**B**) Healing progressed to weight-bearing in 4 months. Both pins were removed at 13 months on an outpatient basis, with a large amount of callus evident at the tibial site. (left, right)

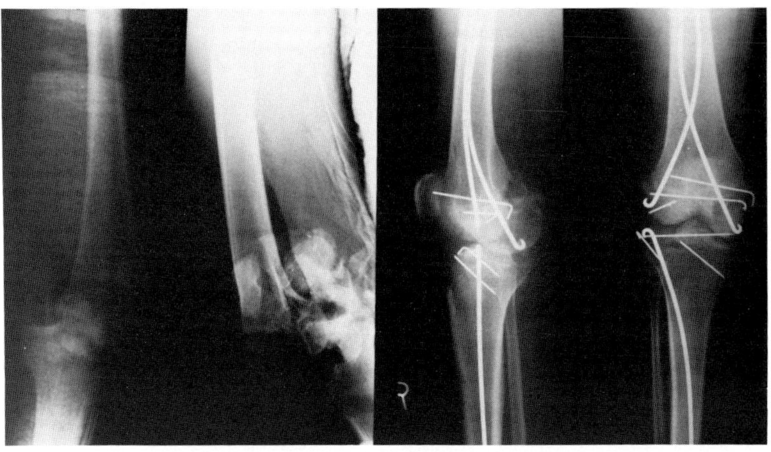

A

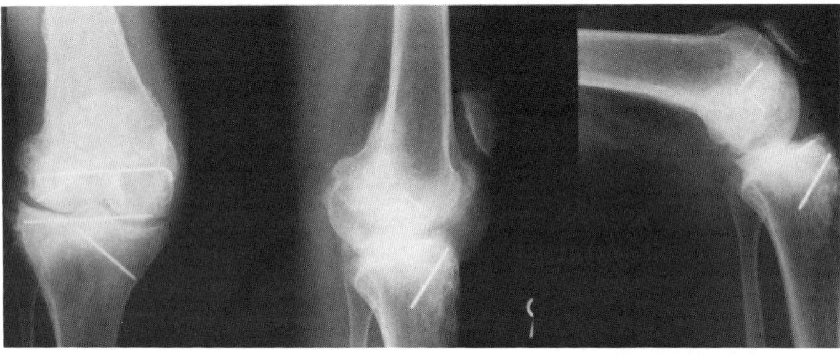

B

Figure 13–4.   Open fractures at the knee joint. (**A**) A 19-year-old woman involved in a motorcycle and car accident suffered an open Gustilo Type III right femoral fracture, with both condyles, both cruciates, partial patella avulsion, complete patellar laceration, tibial plateau, anterior tibial eminence involved, as well as a dislocation of the knee. Immediate debridement and piecemeal pinning of the femoral condyles with straight ⅛-inch (3.18 mm) Rush pins and Kirschner wires was done, and the tibia was pinned with Kirschner wires and ⅛-inch (3.18 mm) straight Rush pins on June 30, 1985. Radiographs were taken at 6 weeks when the wounds had all healed and the skin graft across the patellar tendon was secure. Radiographs were taken on September 6, 1985. (**B**) The patient was started on knee motion, but no weight-bearing until her fractures had united. Radiographs taken on December 28, 1987, after internal fixation devices had been removed, showed range of motion at the knee from 0 to 80 degrees, and the patient was going to college and playing tennis.

SUGGESTED READINGS

Chapman, M.W.: The role of Intramedullary fixation in open fractures. Clin. Orthop. 212:26–34, 1986.

Gustilo, R.B., Anderson, J.T.: Prevention of infection in treatment of one thousand and twenty five open fractures of long bones: retrospective and prospective analysis. J. Bone Joint Surg. 58A:453–458, 1976.

Rittman, W.W., Schibli, M., Matter, P., Allgower, M.: Open fractures: long-term results in 200 consecutive cases. Clin. Orthop. 138:132–140, 1979.

CHAPTER 14

Other Common Fracture Fixation Uses

Clavicle Fracture Technique
Metacarpal Fracture Technique

THE CLAVICLE

The clavicle is infrequently surgically treated as it usually heals by conservative means with a large amount of callus.

Anatomy

The bone is curved in two planes and carries a longitudinal load with rotation of the shoulder and arm. Radiographic control is difficult with only one view usually obtainable. Open treatment is the only safe method of internal fixation because of the proximity of the lungs, great vessels, and neurovascular bundles.

Surgical Treatment

The patient is placed in the supine position with a pad beneath the shoulders (Fig. 14–1). Sterile drapes are applied. An incision along Langer's line is usually possible. The lateral fragment is treated first by inserting the ⅛-inch (3.18 mm) awl reamer into the fracture and going through the posterior distal portion of the clavicle near the acromioclavicular joint. Occasionally a power drill with a bit ⅛ inch (3.18 mm) in diameter, will be needed in young people. The awl reamer is then used to find the lateral hole and the ⅛ inch (3.18 mm) pin is placed across it (Fig. 14–2). This will usually add an additional 2 to 2½ inches (5 to 6 cm) to the length of the pin. The pin is then impacted out through the fracture, the fracture reduced, and the pin inserted so that the hook is near to the cortex.

A ⅛ inch (3.18 mm) pin gives the best fixation and should be long enough to provide fixation. The curved hook prevents medial migration, and because the bone is curved, a straight pin can be used. Fracture healing is easy to evaluate on standard radiographs.

FRACTURE OF THE METACARPALS

In fractures of the metacarpals, the pin is best introduced from the proximal end of the bone. The pin chosen has a ³⁄₃₂

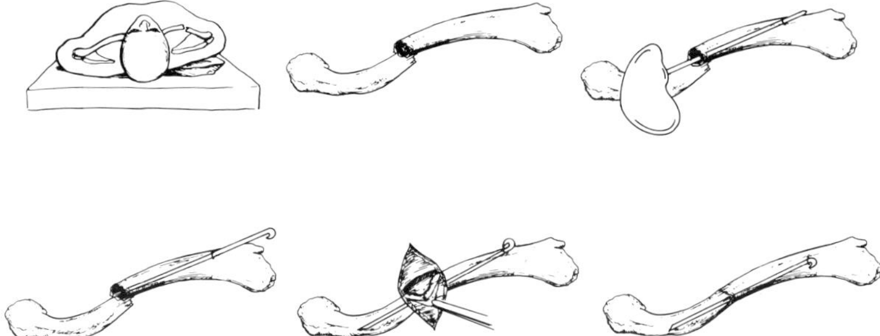

Figure 14–1. Clavicle fractures. Top left to right: Position of a patient for surgery is shown. The fracture is exposed with minimal dissection. One-eighth-inch (3.18 mm) awl reamer or drill is placed out the canal laterally. A pin is placed to the fracture site. The fracture is gently reduced. The pin is inserted down canal, with the sled runner hitting cortex.

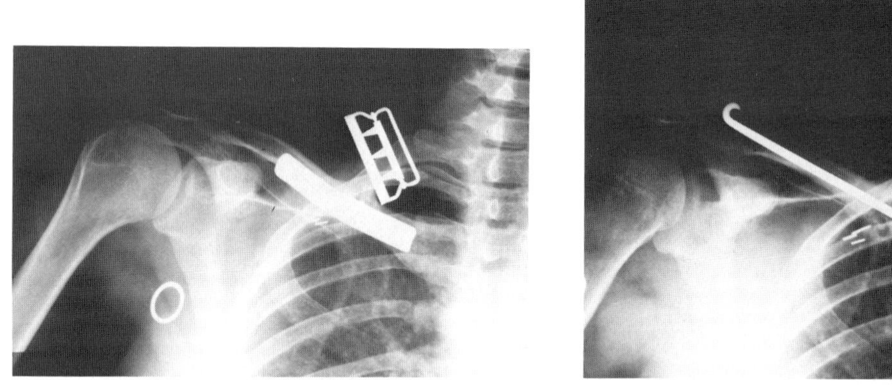

A   B

Figure 14–2. (A) A 23-year-old woman with a severe smoking habit had an avascular limb secondary to an arterial plaque occluding the subclavian artery. A vein graft was applied after the clavicle was split, and it was fixed with a plate and screw fixation. The metal failed at 1 year because the fracture did not heal. (B) At 6 months postoperatively, the plate and screws were removed and a ⅛-inch (3.18 mm) straight Rush pin was inserted along with a bone graft. The patient healed in an additional 4 months.

(2.38 mm) inch diameter and must be meticulously chosen for length. The operation can be carried out in a closed or open procedure. The technique can be greatly simplified by giving the pin a slight curve with the bending iron prior to its insertion.

Through a small stab wound over the dorsum of the proximal and of the metacarpal, an opening is made with the awl reamer as close to the long axis of the bone as possible. The pin is inserted and driven down to the fracture. The reduction is accomplished, and the pin is then driven home so that the point firmly engages the distal fragment. Immediate function can usually be started (Figs. 14–3, 14–4).

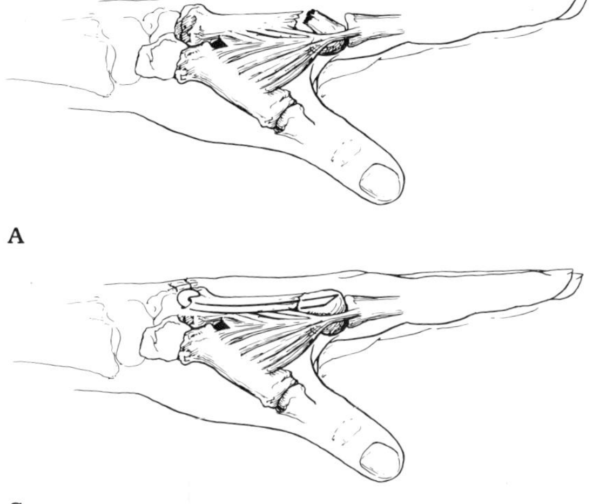

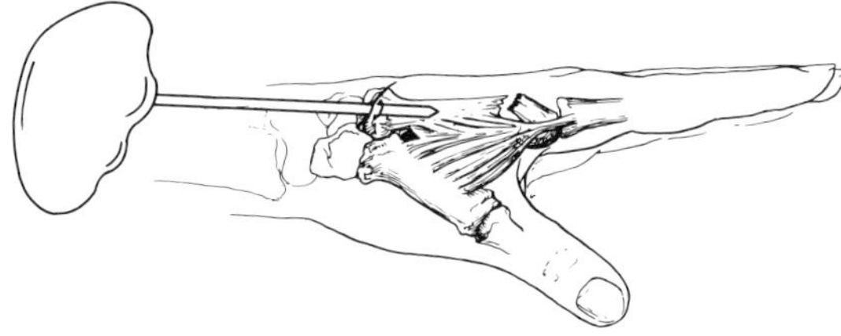

Figure 14–3. (**A**) Displaced fracture of the metacarpal neck is shown. (**B**) The awl is directed into the shaft at the metacarpal base. (**C**) A slightly precurved pin provides good fixation and allows early function.

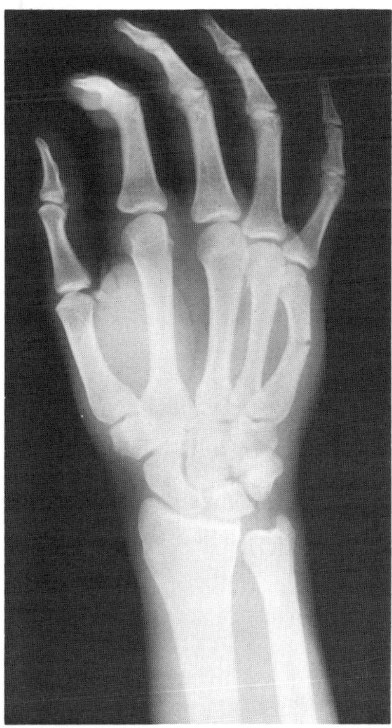

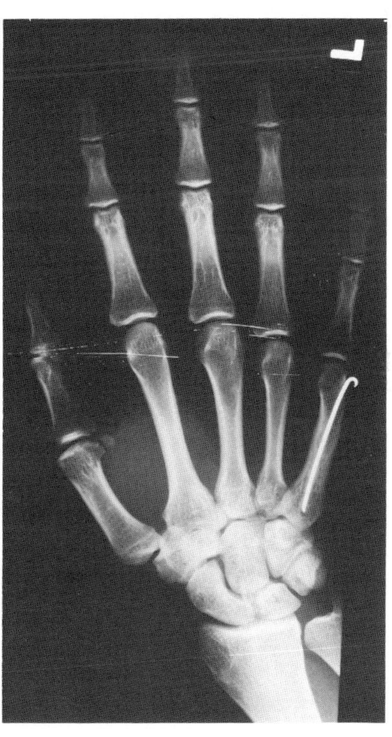

Figure 14–4. (**A**) A 17-year-old boy suffered a fracture of the midshaft of the fifth metacarpal 1 week before a ski trip. (**B**) The fracture was pinned closed, with a $^3/_{32}$-inch (2.38 mm) pin and he went on the ski trip wearing an elastic bandage. Radiographs were taken at 3 months.

Index